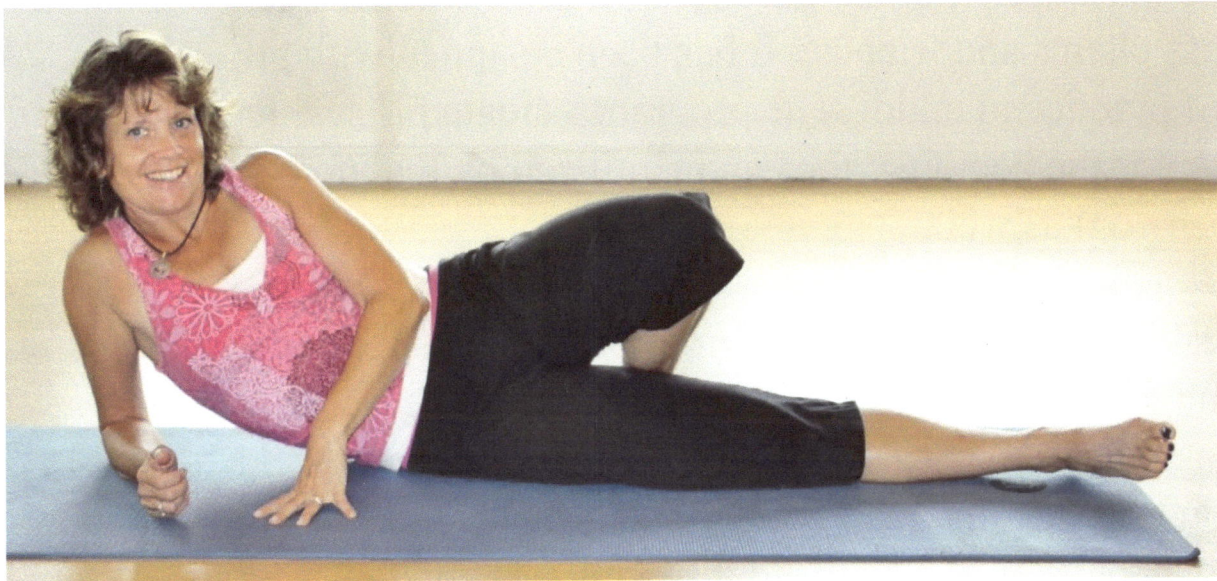

Intro to De Stress

This book is a user-friendly guide for all of my wonderful De Stress clients and friends. It has been designed with all levels of practice in mind. The program I created is safe and effective for the beginner and can be utilized by the more advanced yogi as well.

De Stress is a fusion style program of breathing, stretching, yoga and Pilates. Initially, the emphasis should be on the breath as this is the basis of the mind-body experience. Each time you open this manual, you will simply need to decide what your focus or goal is for that session. Then integrate the breath with your practice and allow the chosen grouping of asanas to inspire your workout.

Requirements

A great mind set or desire to achieve one!

A yoga mat or nonslip surface. A carpet or rug would also be suitable. If a less strenuous workout is desired, the asanas may be done with a chair.

Comfortable attire is always suggested. Unrestrictive clothing or sports wear will allow ease of movement and breathing.

I prefer bare feet but know that some clients are more comfortable in some kind of foot covering. Socks may not allow for gripping and shoes may be bulky, so you decide what will work best for your practice.

You will also be utilizing your CORE and Chakras. I will briefly discuss each term in order to make you more aware of these integral parts of your body.

The Core

The core is located at your abdominal area. It is defined as the region bound by the abdominal wall, pelvis, lower back and diaphragm. You will utilize this area throughout your movements and breathing. With practice you will learn how to link the two together. The diaphragm is the primary muscle for breathing and is essential for providing the necessary core stability for moving through your De Stress program.

The lower back or lumbar spine is also responsible for posture stability and strength that will enhance your practice.

Chakras

The CHAKRAS span from the crown of your head down to the base of the abdomen. They are the seven main energy centers of the body. These energy spirals each relate to one another and help to unite the mind, body and spirit in a Holistic manner. It may help you to imagine these energy centers as wheels that spin and connect to one another as you lift your breath and energy through your body.

When we begin the breathing process, you will work from the lowest chakra engaging your core and lifting the oxygen up through the energy spirals to the top chakra or crown. The breath will also move through the spine. This will help you to sit up tall as your chest and shoulders open along with your mind. Not only will you be seated more erectly but mental clarity and focus will become sharper. Now, you are ready to embrace your practice and truly De Stress.

Chakras

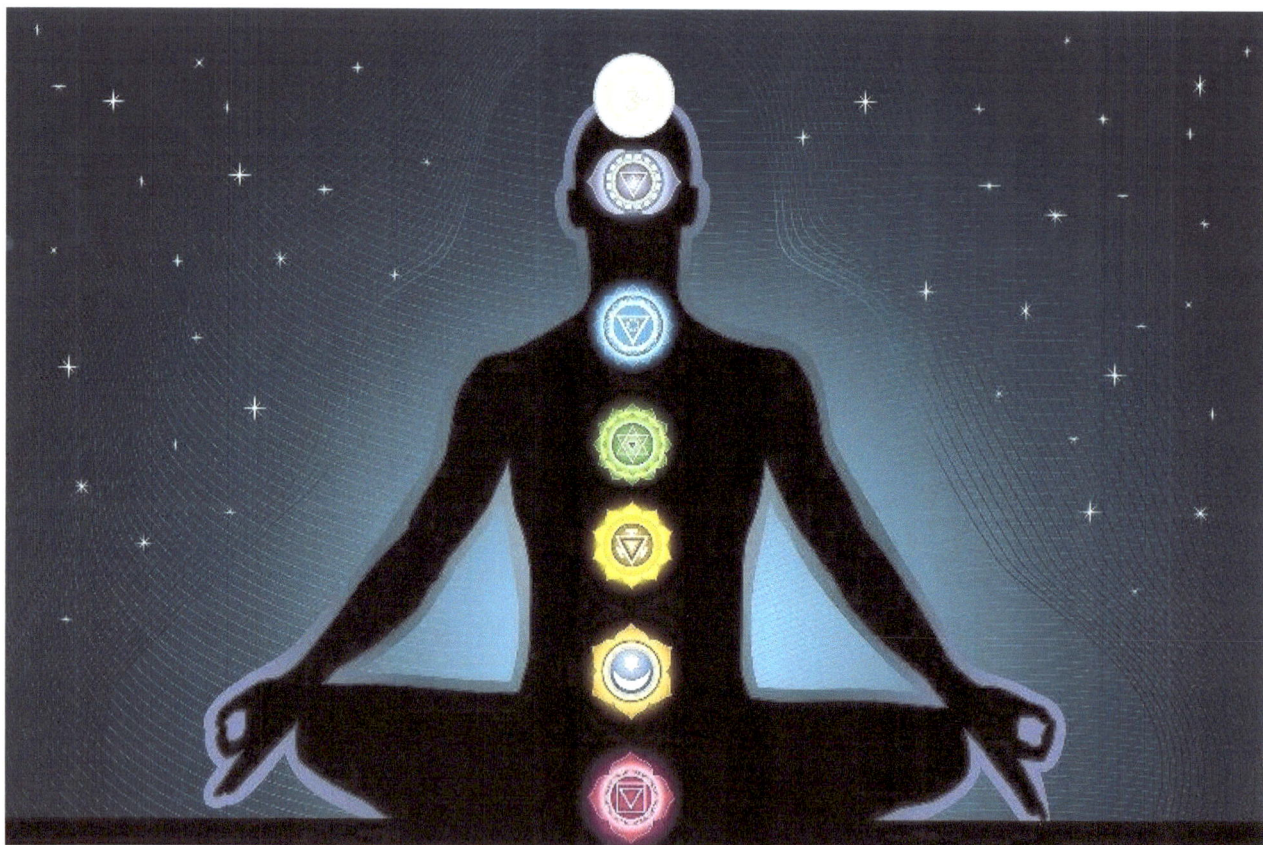

De Stress Breathing

The breathing can be the most challenging part of your practice. Embrace what you can do at the beginning and as you grow with your practice, this involuntary process will change the state of your mind and body.

The breath that I recommend is the Ujjayi, also known as the "ocean" breath. There are three compelling reasons for this choice. The first, is the sound it creates. The second, is the visual effect. When embraced properly, you may be able to hear and visualize the ocean. The third and most powerful reason, is the impact this has on the parasympathetic nervous system. This technique slows down the heart and breathing rates. It also has the potential to lower your blood pressure. Ultimately, this allows you to achieve calmness and De Stress.

I suggest starting in a comfortable seated position or asana. If possible, begin in the Lotus pose, the first asana shown in this manual. Your hands may be down if you are feeling grounded or palms up so that you remain open to the entire process and receive energy.

Another option would be to find a very comfortable place and lay down in a supine position. Relax your legs and arms and close your eyes. Again, your hand placement can be palms up or down. Gently elongate your neck as you soften your face and allow your cheek bones to relax.

You will begin with a deep inhalation through your nose, becoming aware of the breathing process and how you are feeling. Inhale positive energy as you clear your mind and focus only on your breath. The exhalation will also be through your nose utilizing the muscles in your throat. This will create that "ocean" sound and perhaps a visual as the oxygen moves in and out of your body.

In either position you want to breathe into your abdomen or CORE. If you are lying down, you may want to place your hands at your CORE area while you guide your breath in and out of your lungs. Repeat the process several times without rushing as you become more aware that your mind and body are slowing.

Once you become comfortable with this breath or your own breathing pattern, you will be able to unite your mind and body for your De Stress session.

Each Asana or pose you see in this manual will have a breath attached to the movement. The movements will synch to the breath and the two will intertwine as you move through your session.

Each page will offer asanas, as well as modifications. This will allow you to work at your own level and advance as you become more familiar with your own practice and your goals change.

Your De Stress Practice

Your first sessions may utilize a smaller grouping of asanas so you can become more comfortable with your breath and the mind body experience. Your preference of poses may be determined by the amount of time you have to dedicate to your practice. In order to achieve your goals you should incorporate a realistic amount of time so you may truly embrace where you are on any given day.

Ultimately, you want to move through the entire sequence of the book.

Indoor or Outdoor

You may also choose to take your practice outside so that you can soak up the beauty and benefits of being in nature. Studies have shown that spending as little as five minutes in a natural setting can increase your mood and self-esteem.

De Stress Terminology

ASANA - pose or De Stress position

CHAKRA - energy spirals or wheels

CHI - energy created through your practice

CORE - abdominal area

DRISHTI - focal point to place your visual energy

HEART CENTER - midway up on your Chakras

UJJAYI - Ocean breath

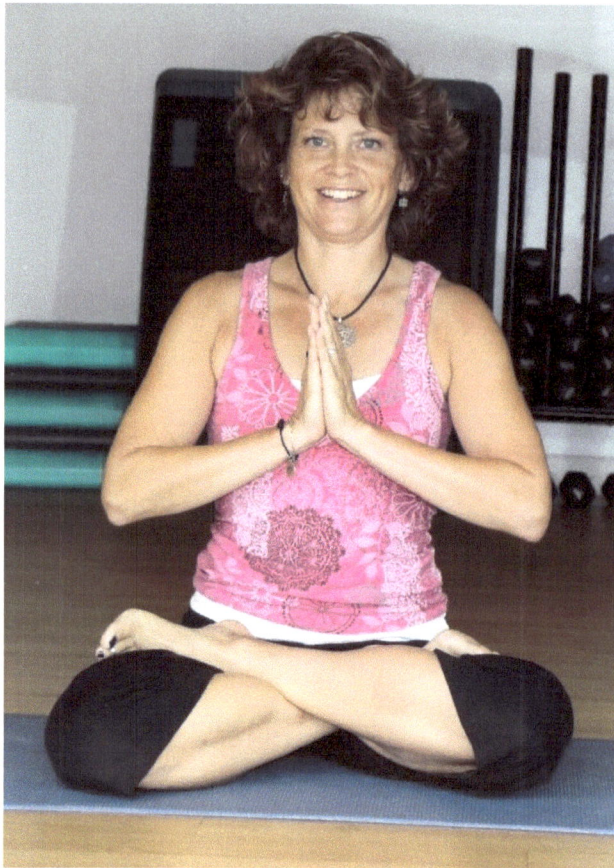

Lotus Hands
in Prayer
At Hearts Center

Lotus Palms Up
to Receive

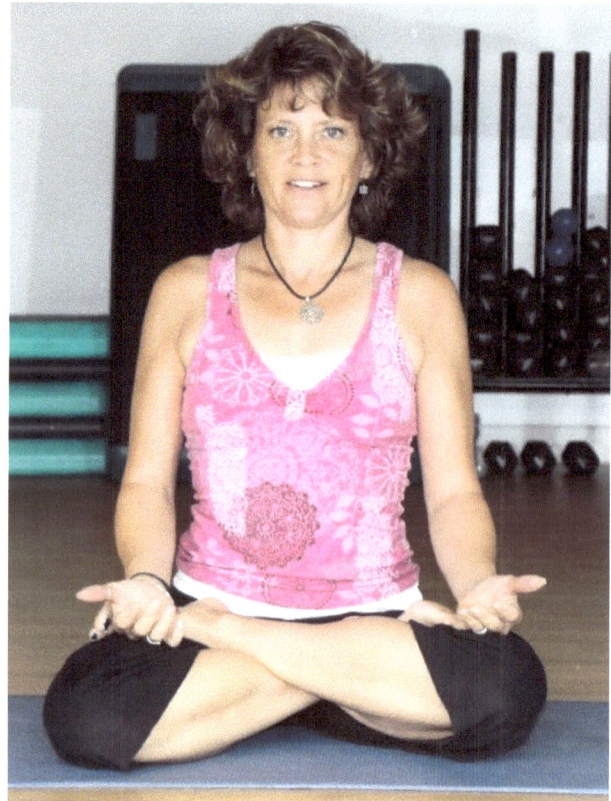

**Begin
Seated**

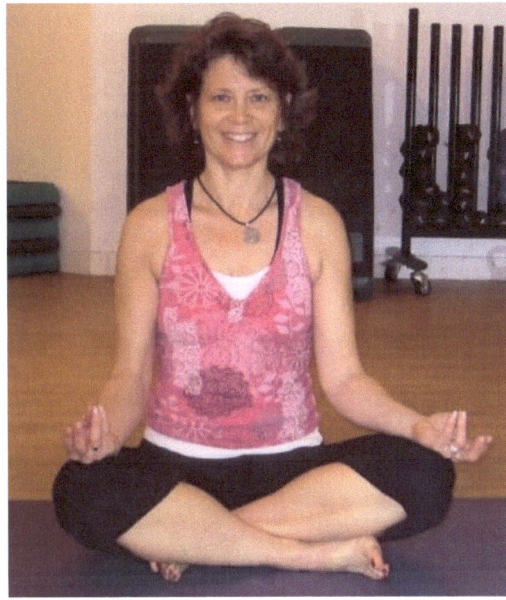

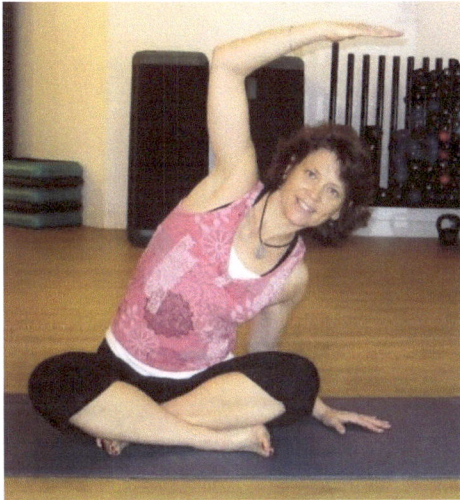

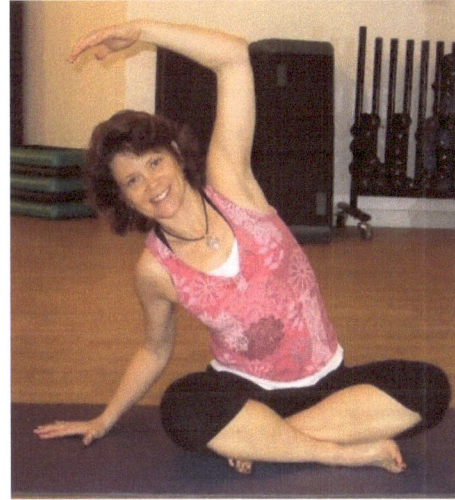

**Side Stretch to the
Left Then
to the Right**

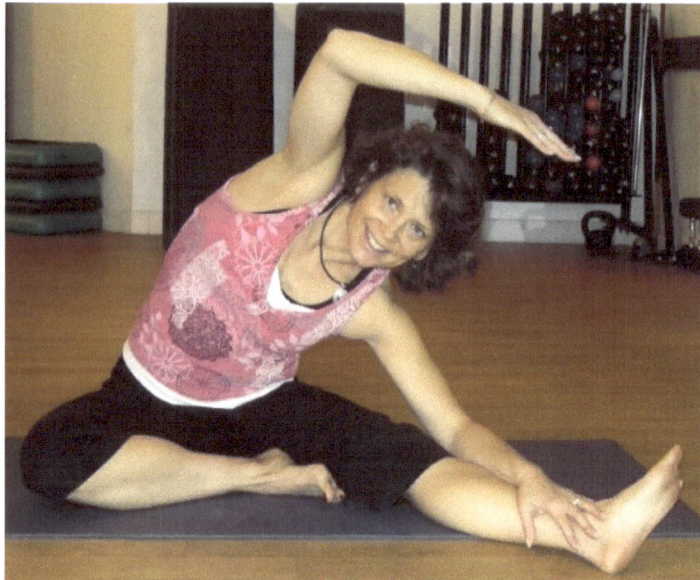

Seated Left Side Stretch with Oblique Rotation

Kick Back on Right Side

Hand Centered under Right Shoulder

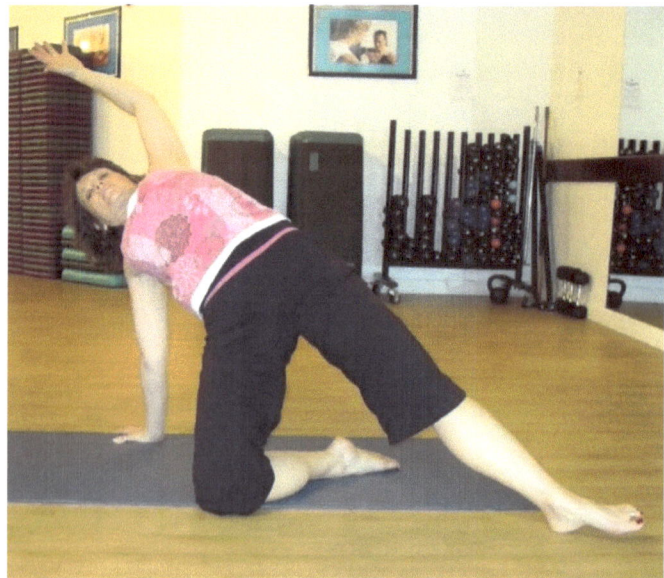

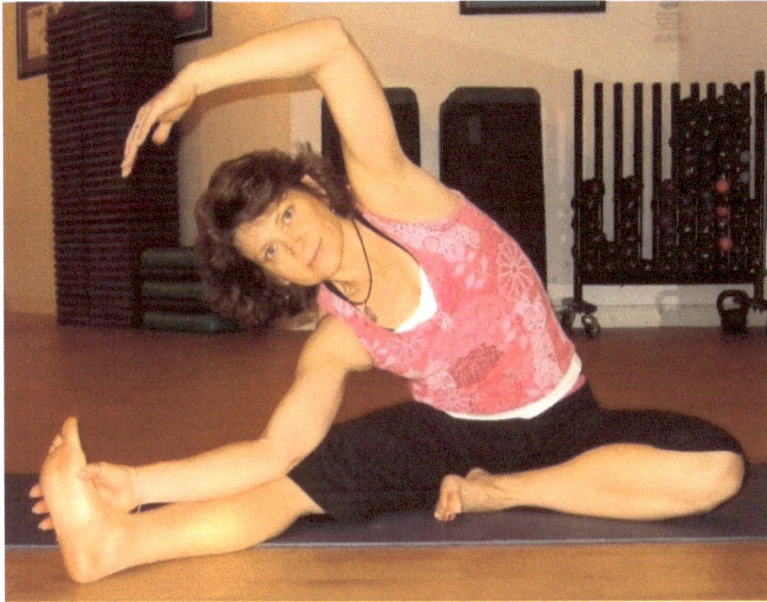

Seated Right Side Stretch with Oblique Rotation

Kick Back on Left Side

Hand Centered under Left Shoulder

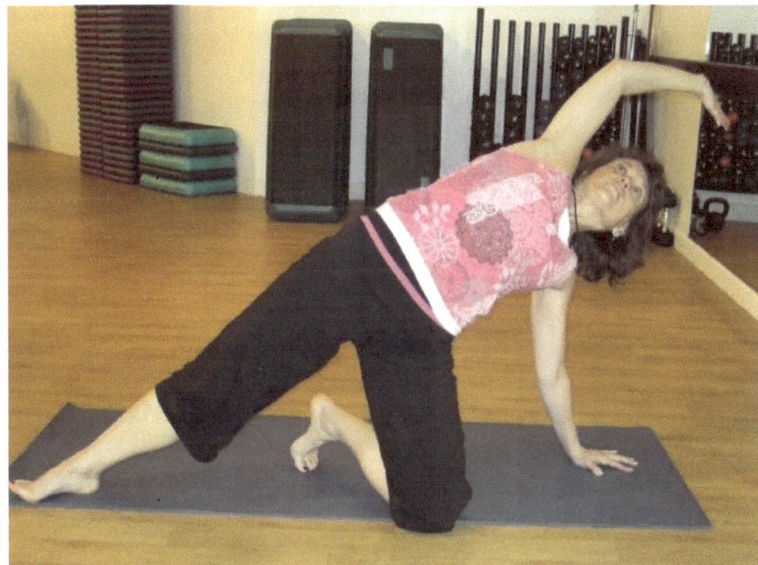

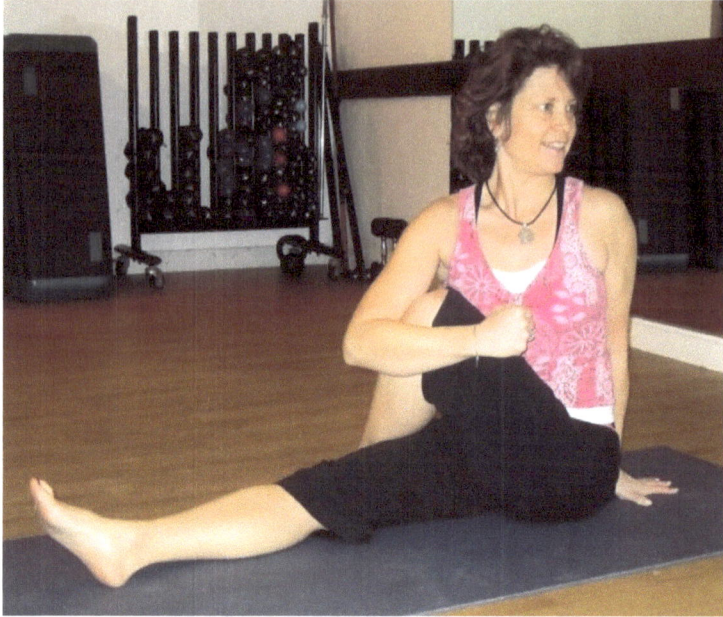

Seated Left Spinal Twist

Wrap Right Arm Around Left Leg and Tuck Belly Button In

When Asana Complete, Do the Right Side

Wrap Left Arm Around Right Side

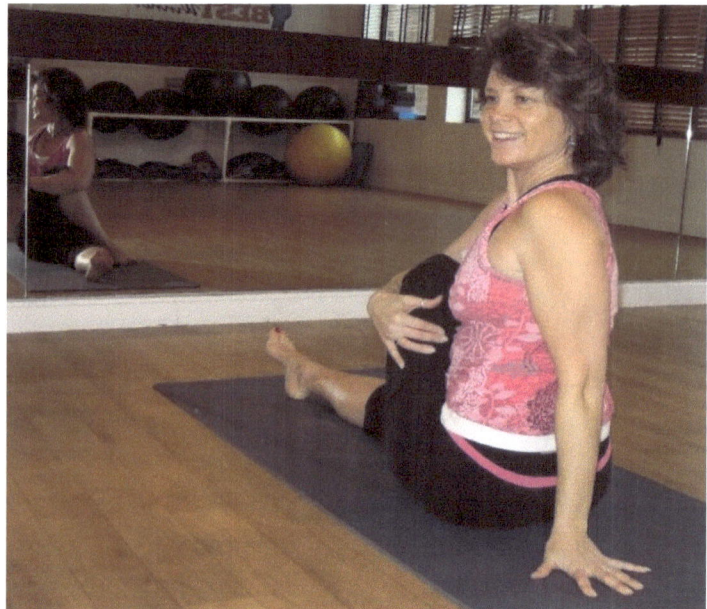

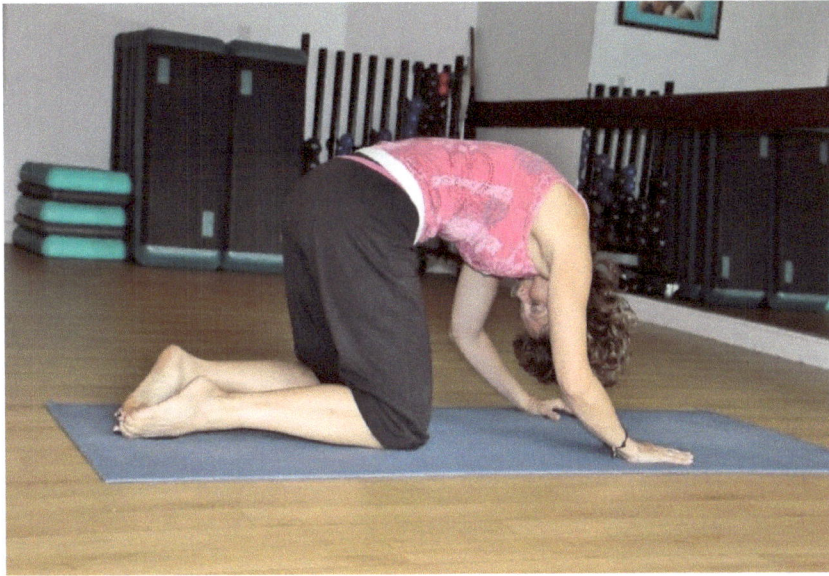

Cat

Tuck Belly Button into Spine and Round Back

Cow

Release Belly Button Lift Crown of Head with Tail to the Sky

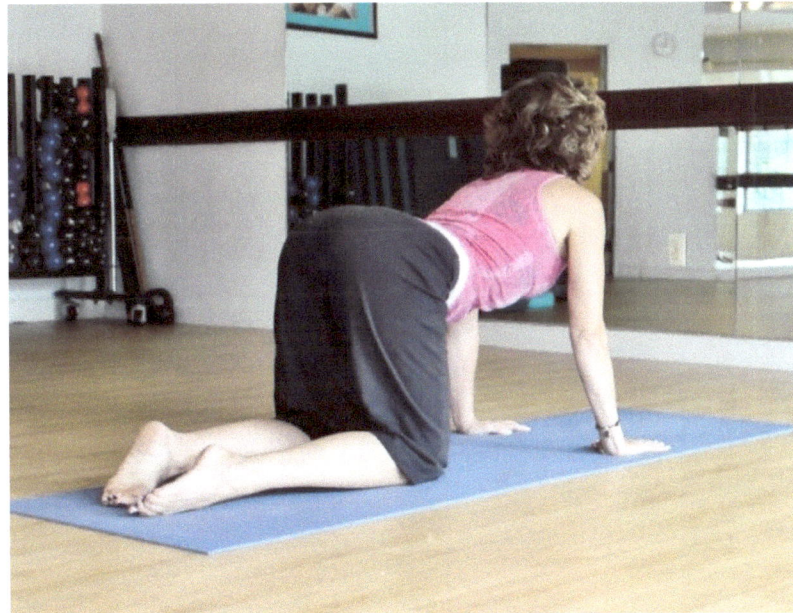

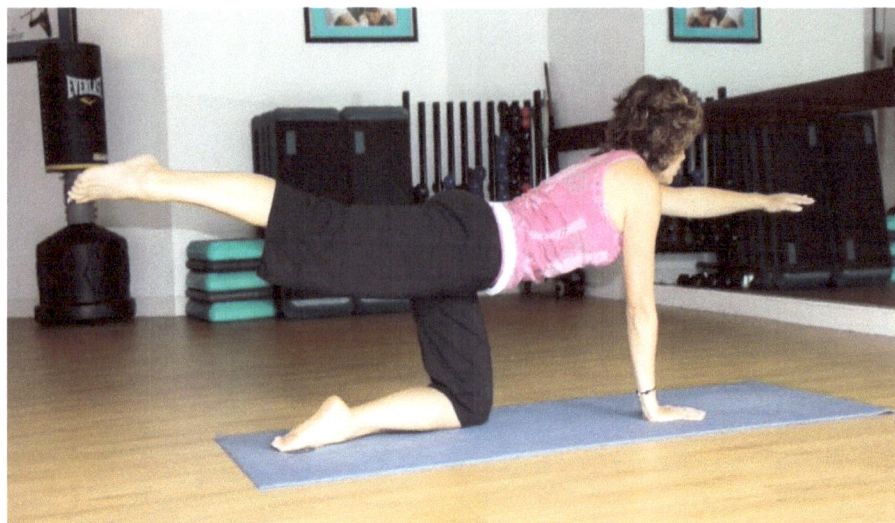

Kneeling Dancer

Kneeling Dancer with Hand Wrapped to Ankle

Repeat on Your Other Leg

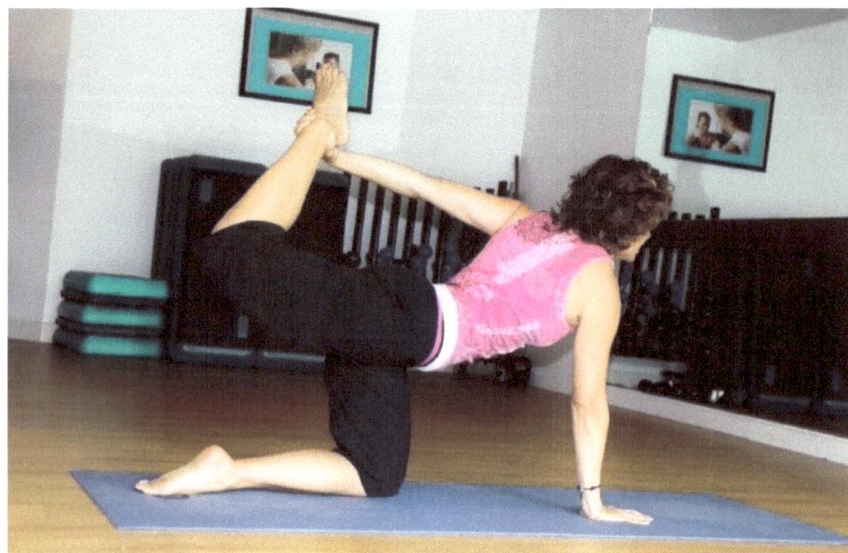

Child's Pose

Tuck Belly Button In and Roll Back Onto Knees with Crown of Head to Earth

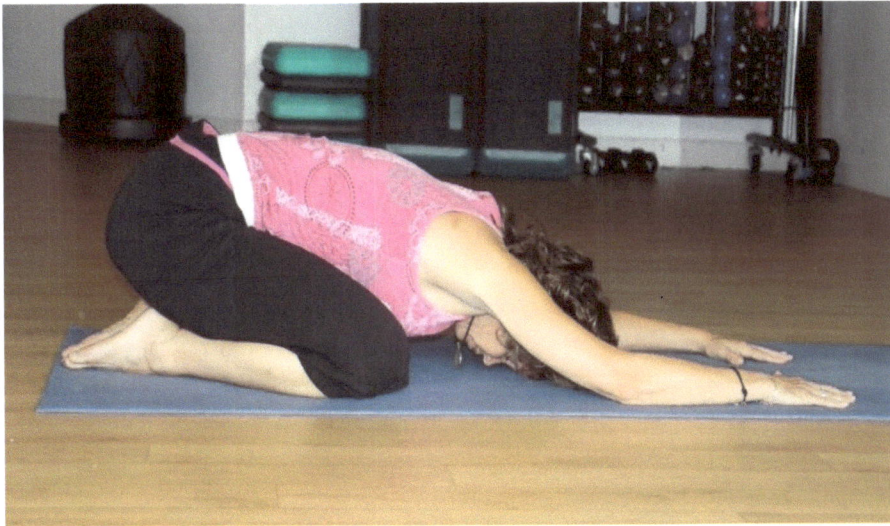

Child's Pose with Arms Wrapped

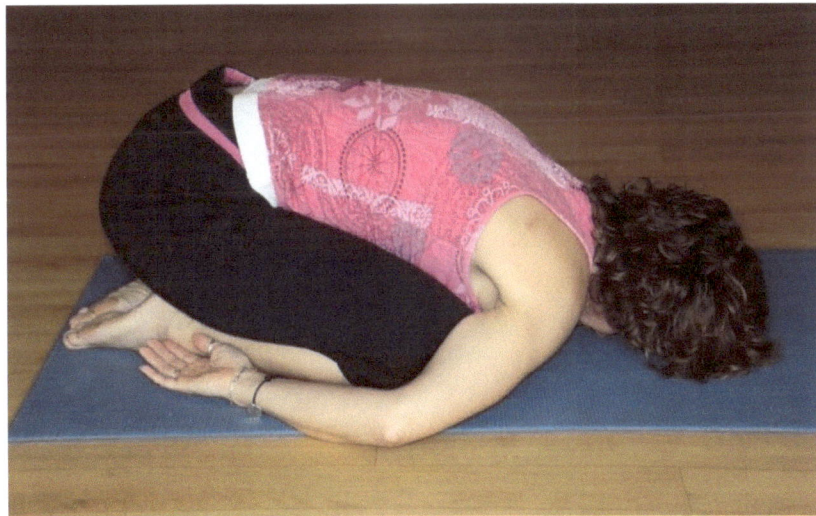

Full Plank

Tuck Belly Button into Spine with Flat Back

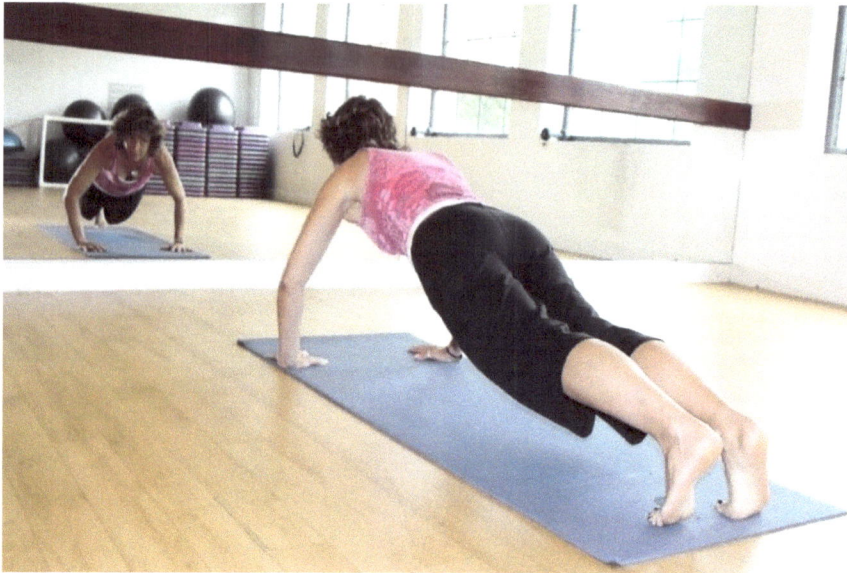

Plank on Elbows

Flat Back with Belly Button Tucked In

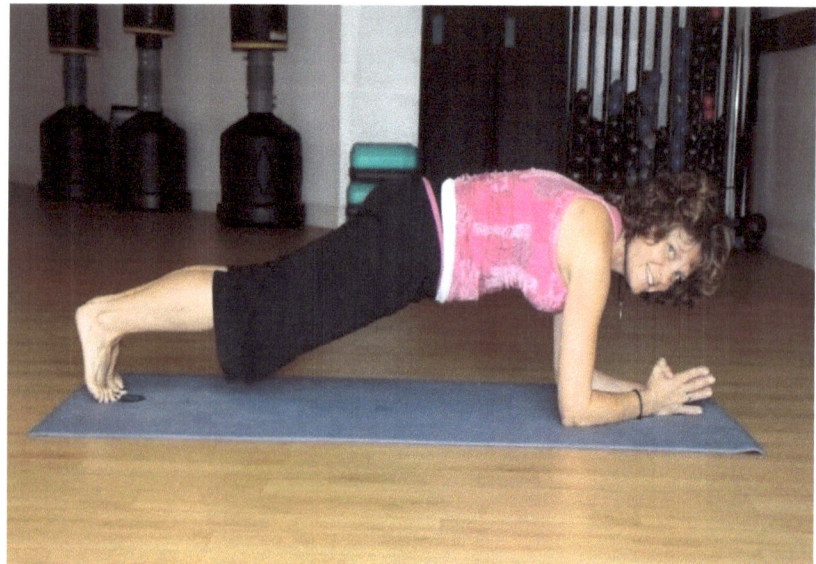

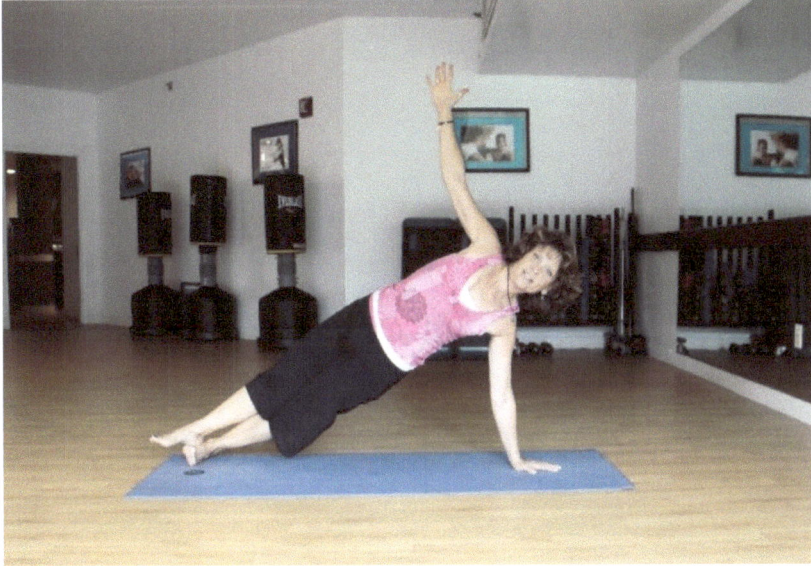

Side Plank

Need to repeat on other side

Side Plank with Leg Extension

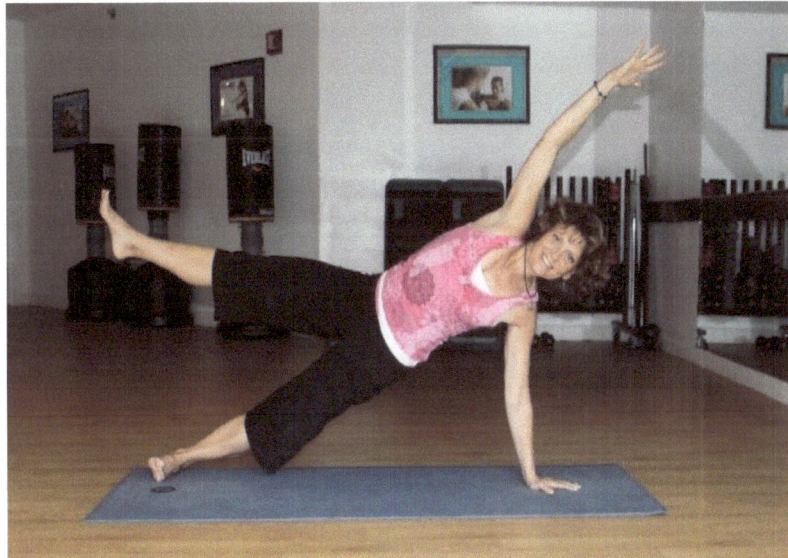

Full Plank

Pull your belly button into your spine

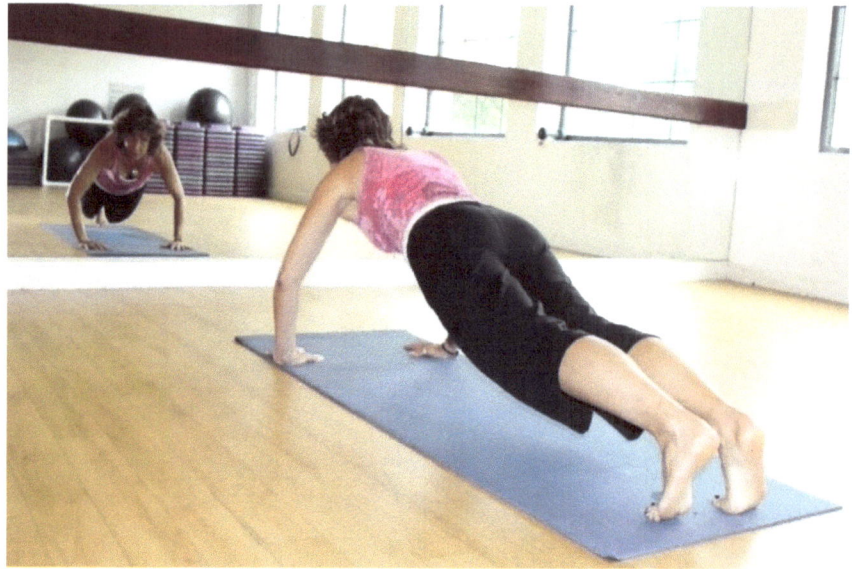

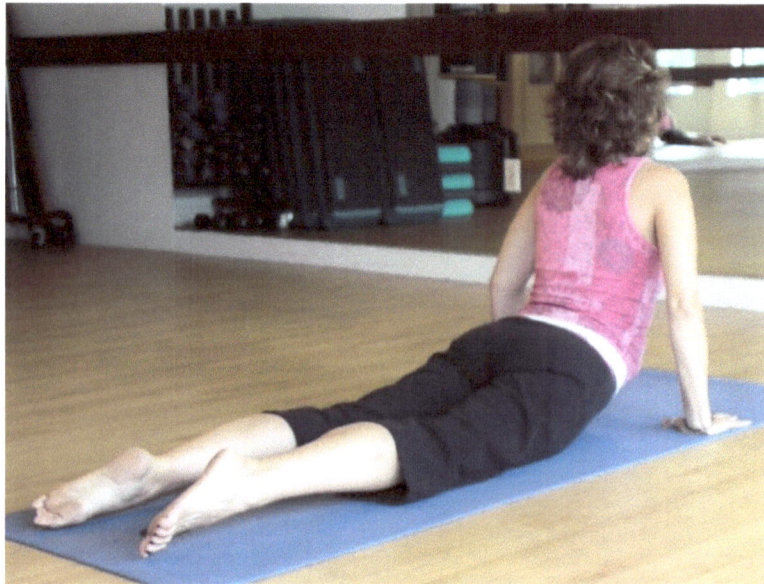

Cobra

Open Chest with Elbows Bent while You Pull Belly Button In

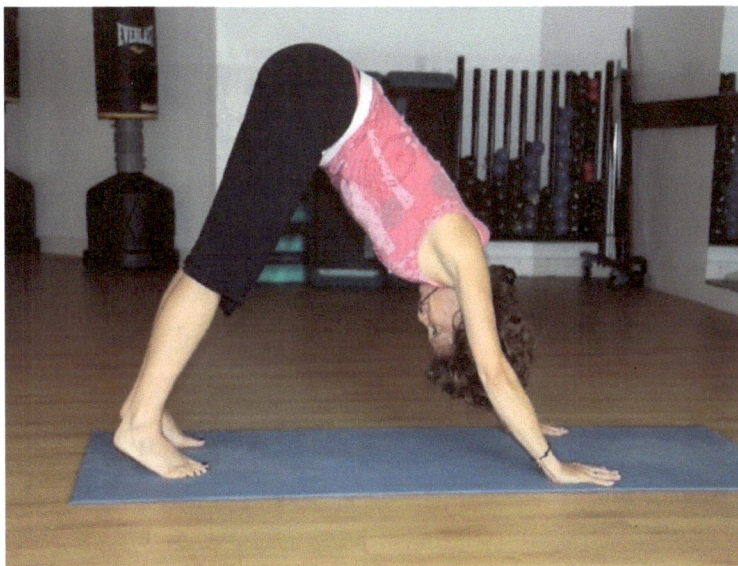

Down Dog

**Tuck Belly
Button in, Lift
Tail to Sky and
Lower Heels
Towards Earth**

Three Legged
Dog

**Lift One Leg at a
Time to the Sky with
Chest Open and Lifting
to the Sky**

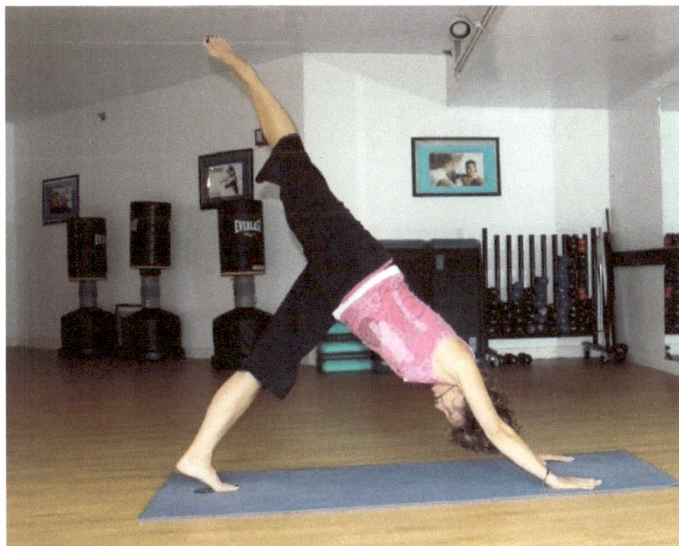

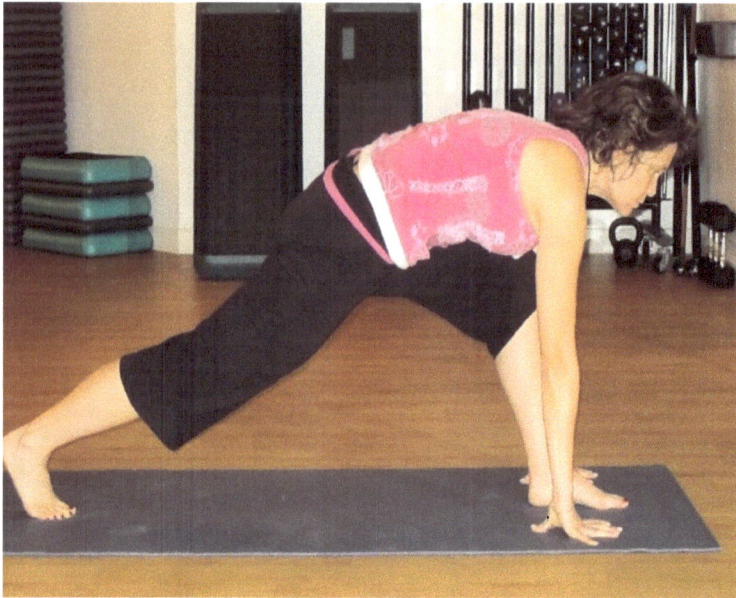

Lunge

Left Foot Should be Under Left Knee

Lunge with a Twist

Complete on Each Side

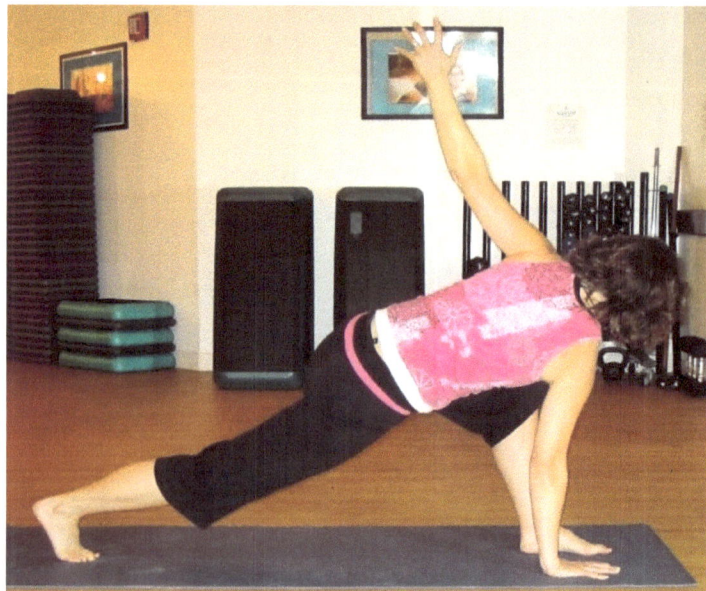

Warrior 1
on Left Side

**Lift Arms to Sky with
Chest Open
Pull Right Hip Forward
and Left Hip Back with
Belly Button Tucked In**

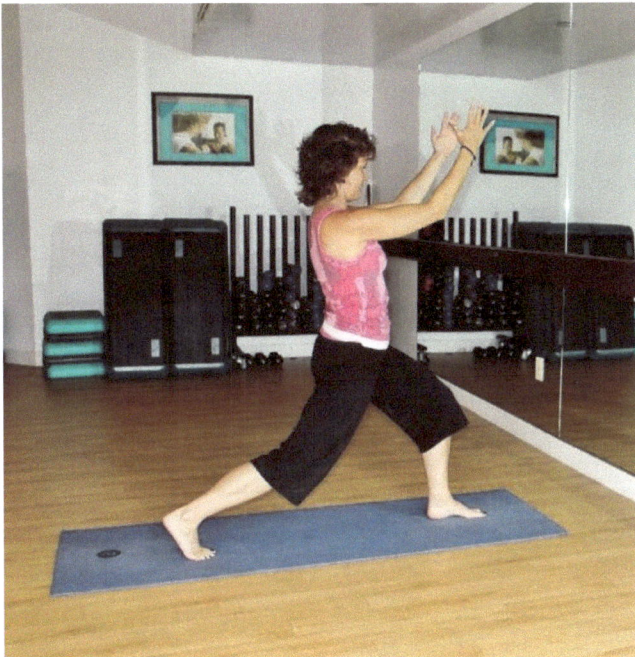

Rotate into
Warrior 2

**Left Arm Will Be Extended
Forward to Front of Mat and
Right Arm Extended Back**

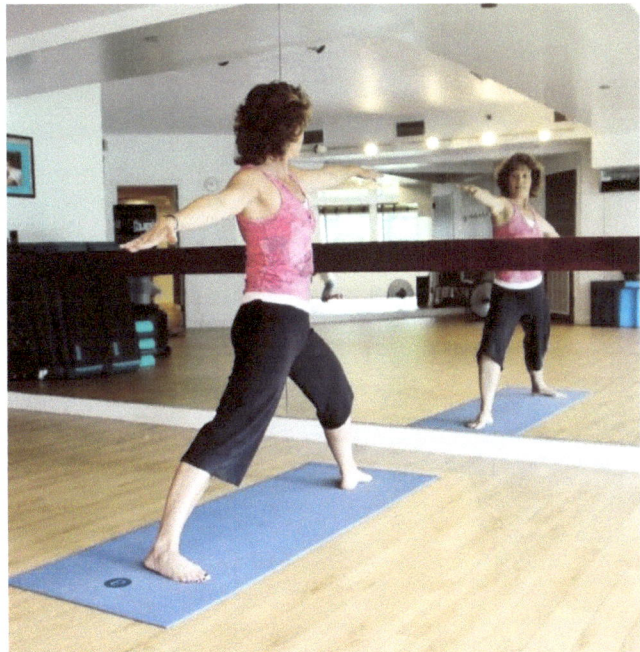

Warrior 1 on Right Side

**Lift Arms to the Sky
Open the Chest
Pull Left Hip Forward
and Right Hip Back with
Belly Button Tucked In**

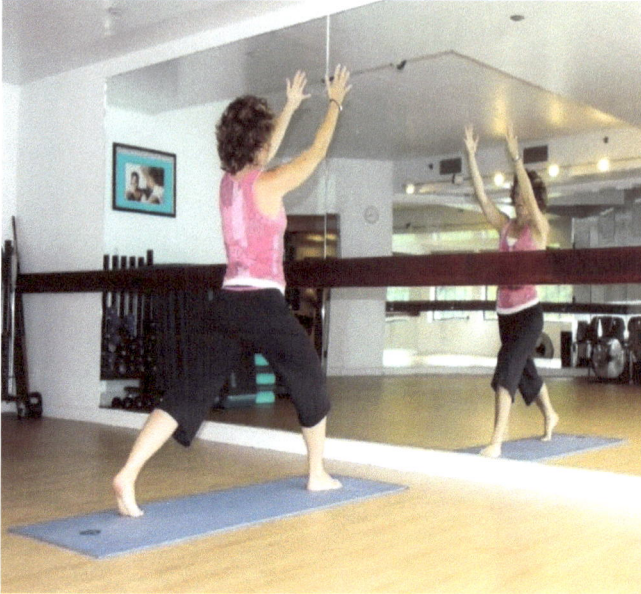

Rotate into Warrior 2

**Right Arm Will Be
Extended Forward
To the Front of Mat and
Left Arm Extended
Back**

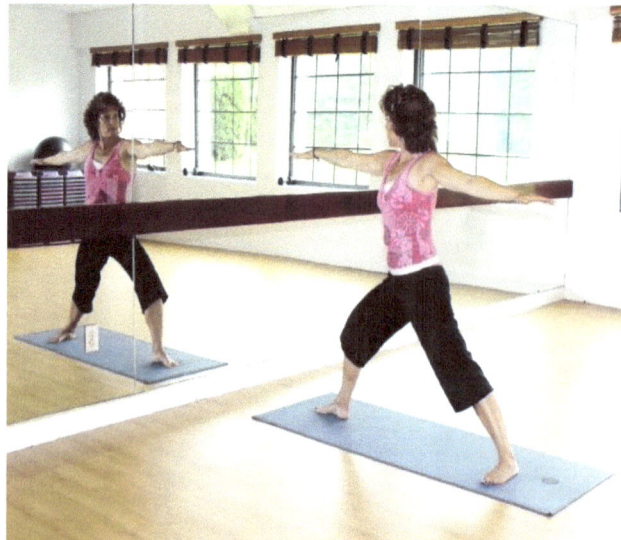

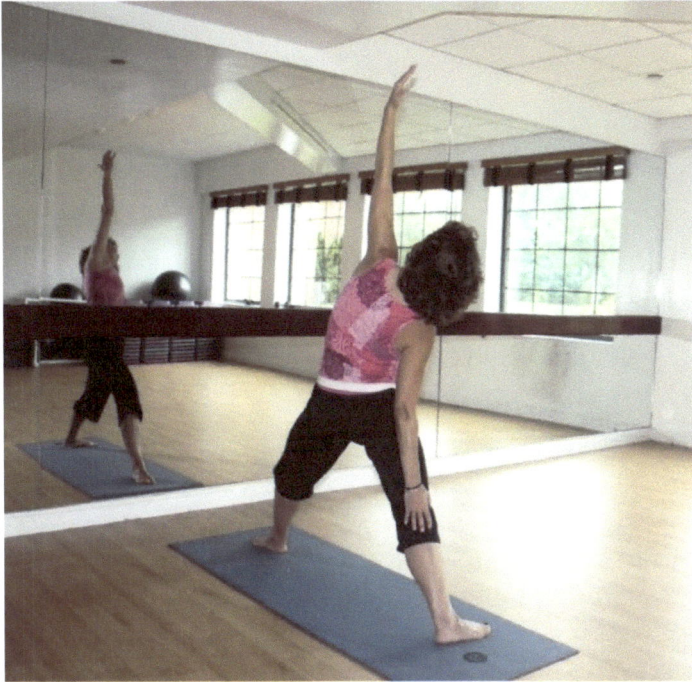

Reverse Warrior

Rotate Back on Straight Leg and Extend Opposite Arm to the Sky

Side Angle

Fold Onto Front Bent Leg and Extend Opposite Arm to Sky

Complete on Each Side

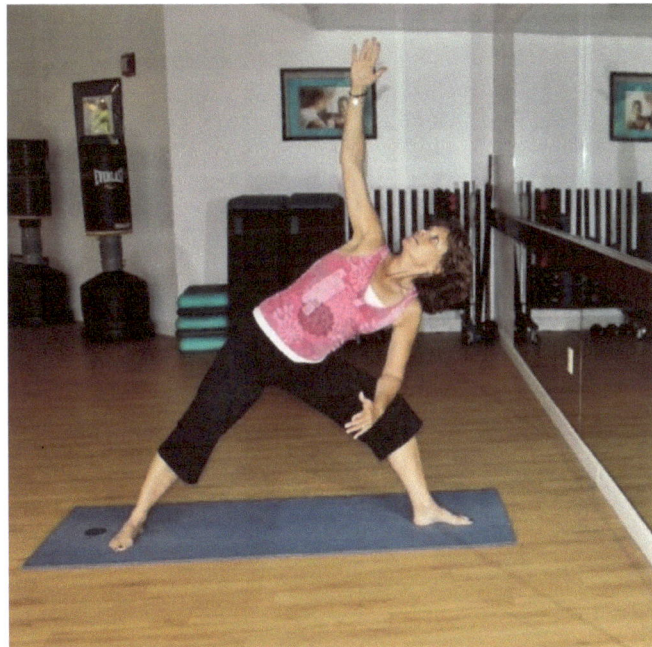

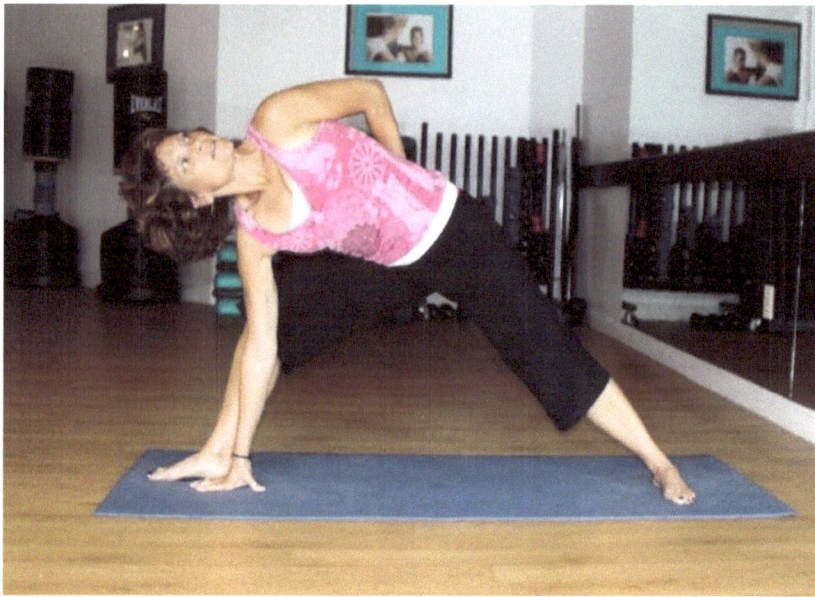

Left Arm Wraps on to Lower Back

Bound Angle

Right Arm Tucks Under Right Leg to Work to the Left Hand

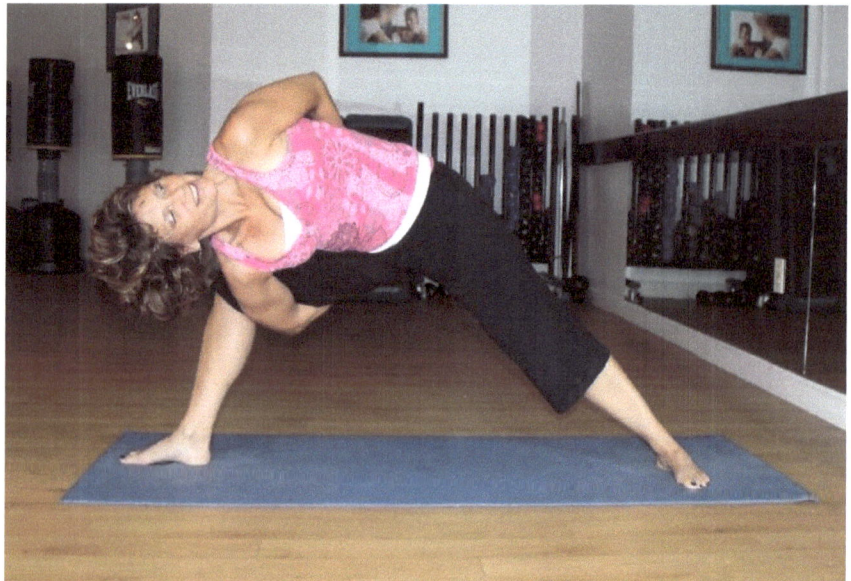

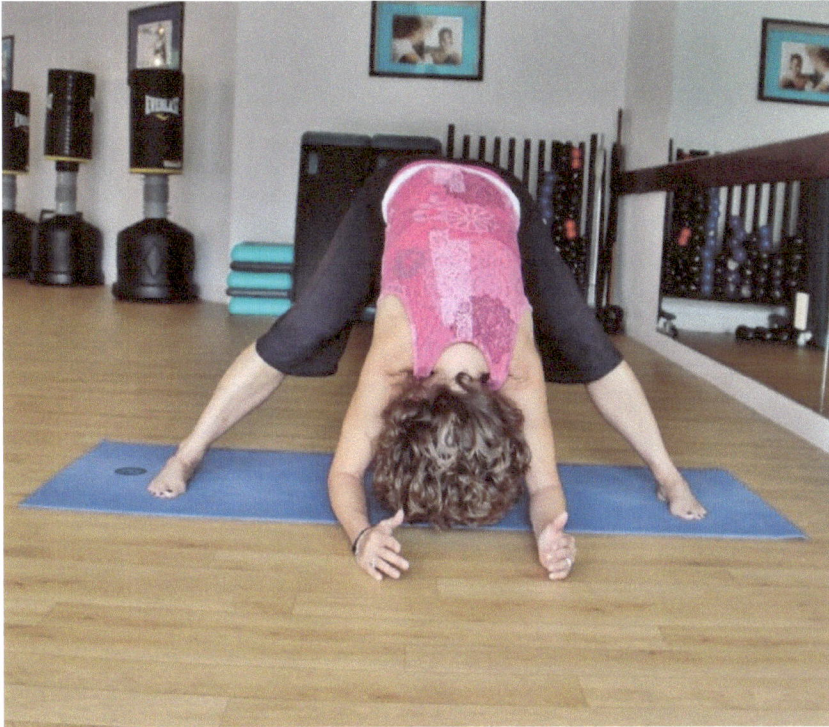

Bring It Center & Breathe

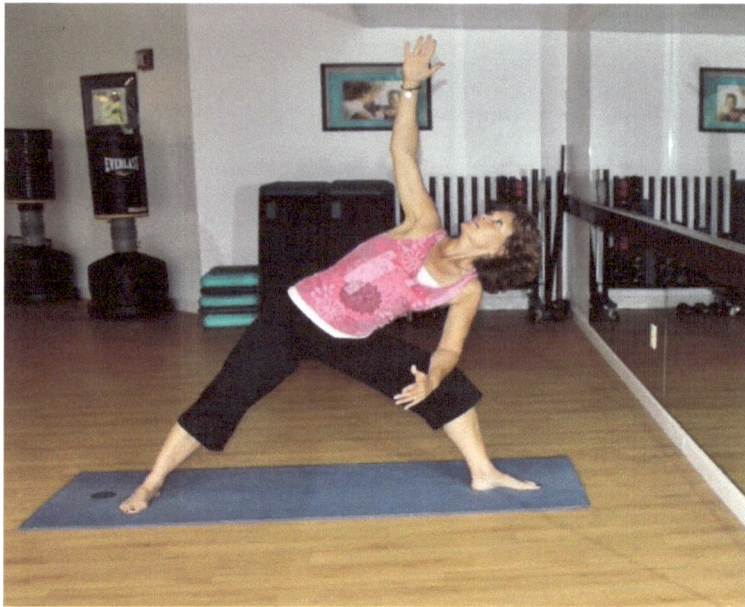

Right Arm Wraps on to Lower Back

Bound Angle

Left Arm Tucks Under Left Leg to Work to the Right Hand

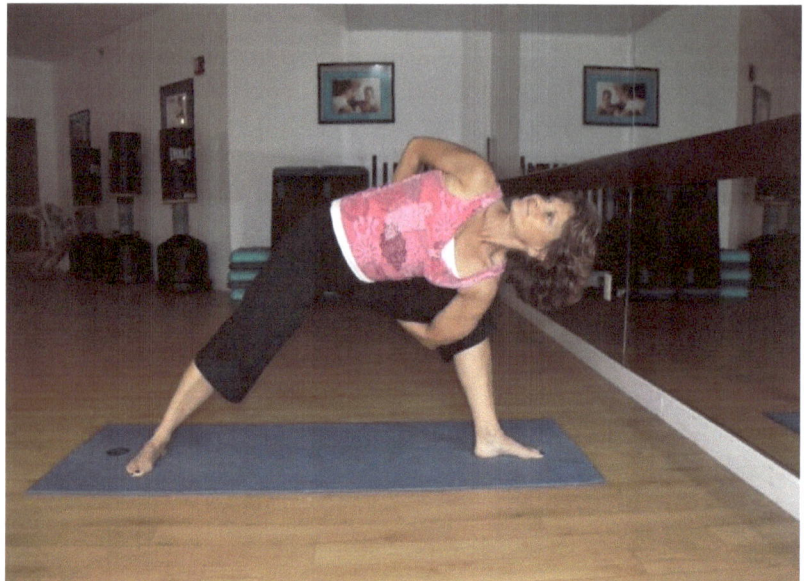

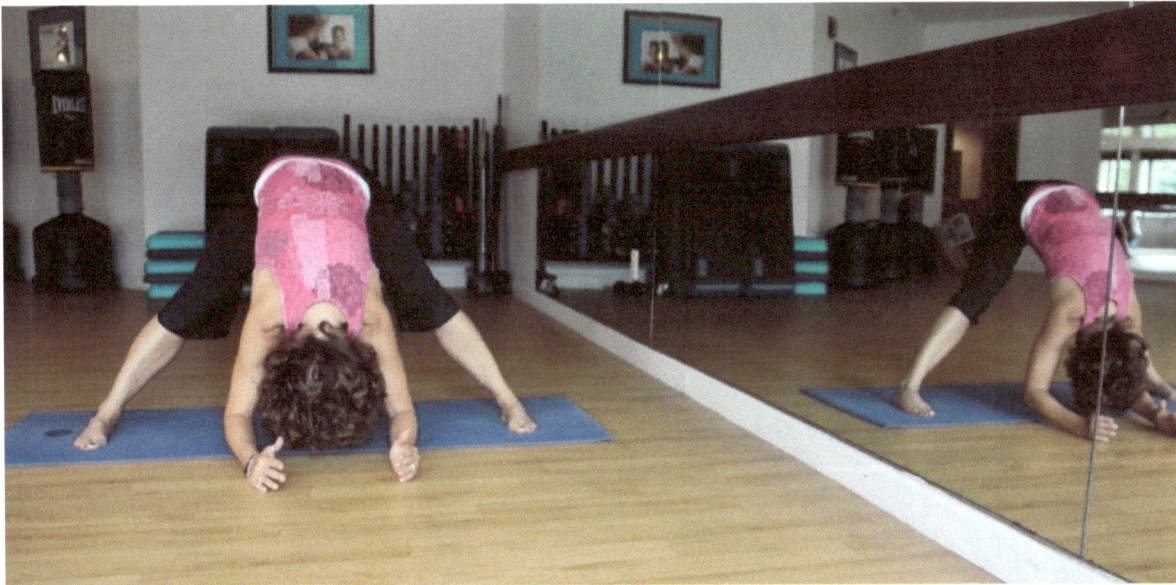

Take it to Center

Lower Your Head to the Earth with Your Inhale

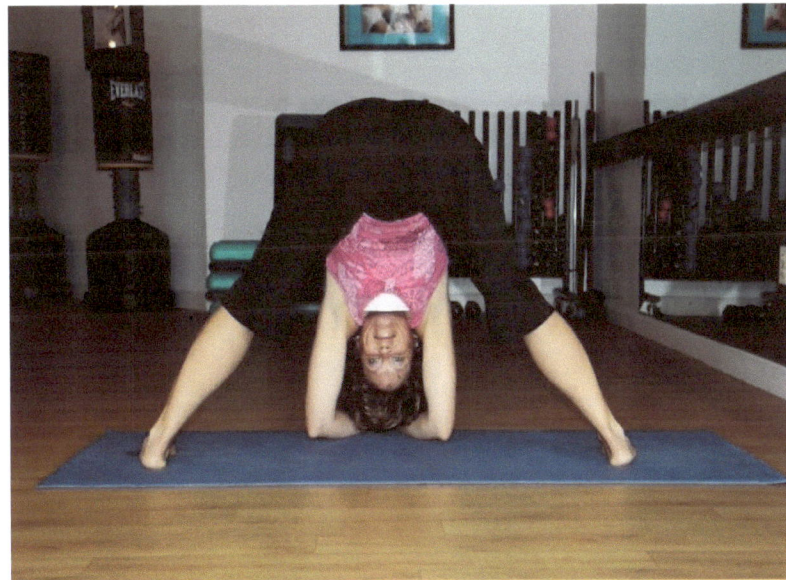

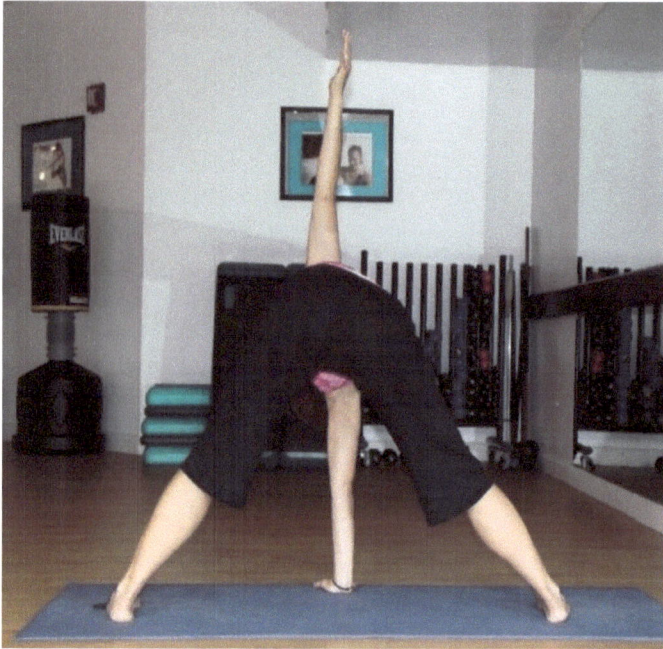

Center Right Hand & Twist with Left Arm to the Sky

Center Left Hand & Twist Right Arm to the Sky

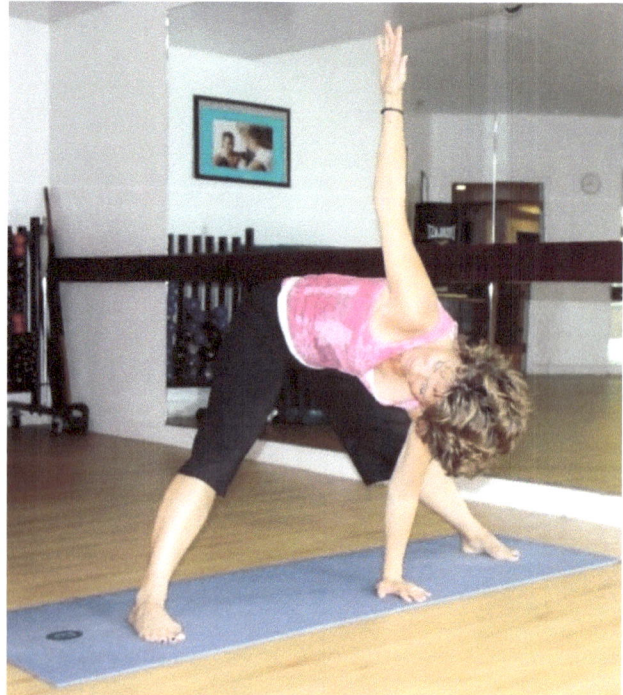

Full Plank

Pull Belly Button into Spine with Back Straight

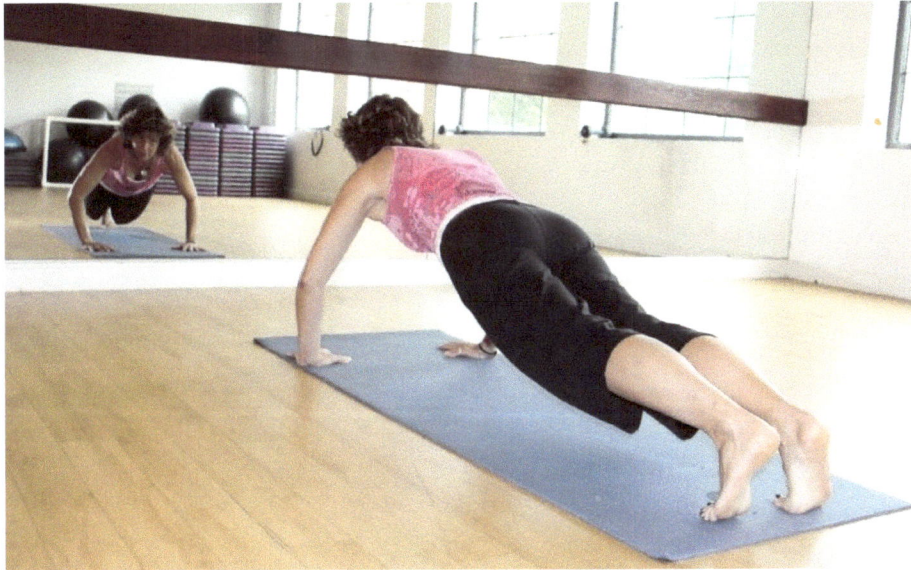

To Hover

This Can Be Done with Knees on the Floor

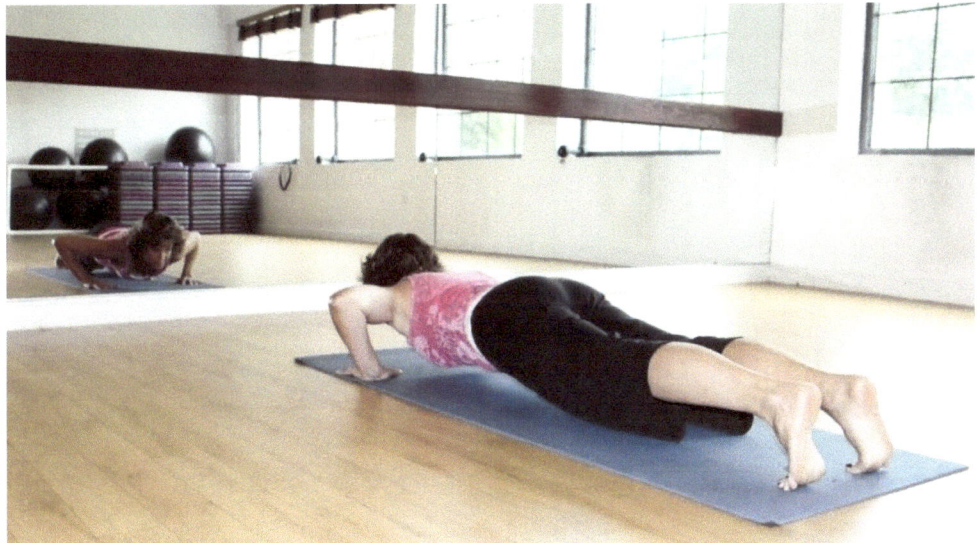

Super Man

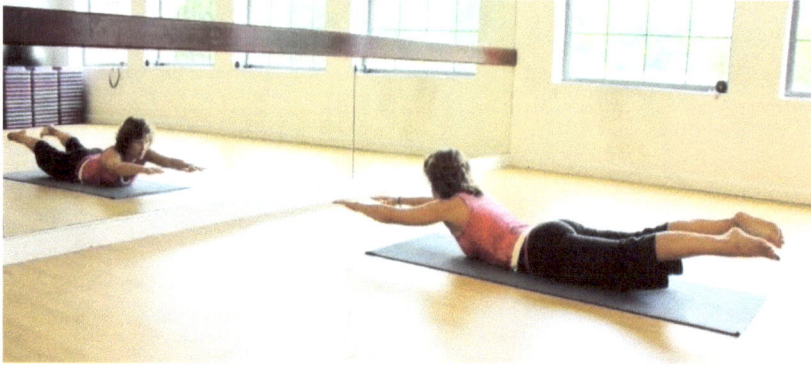

Pull from Your Center
Extending Arms & Legs

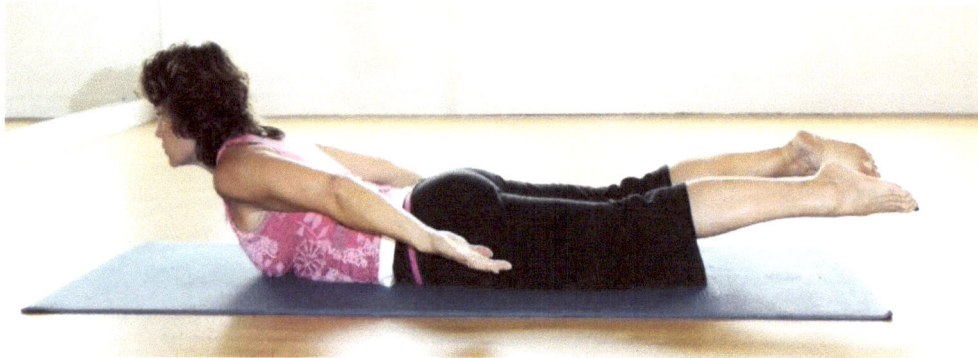

Super Woman

Open Chest as You Extend Arms Back

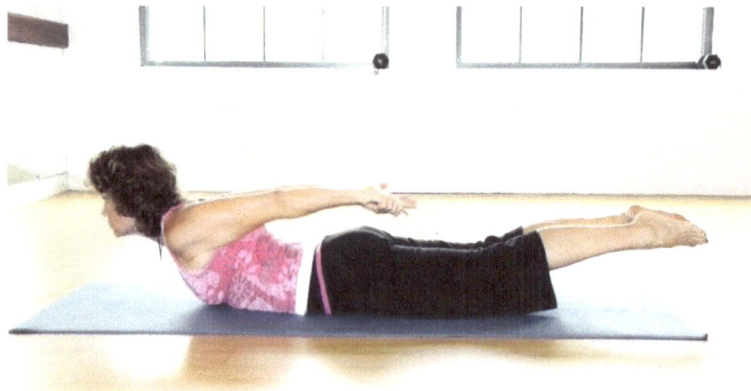

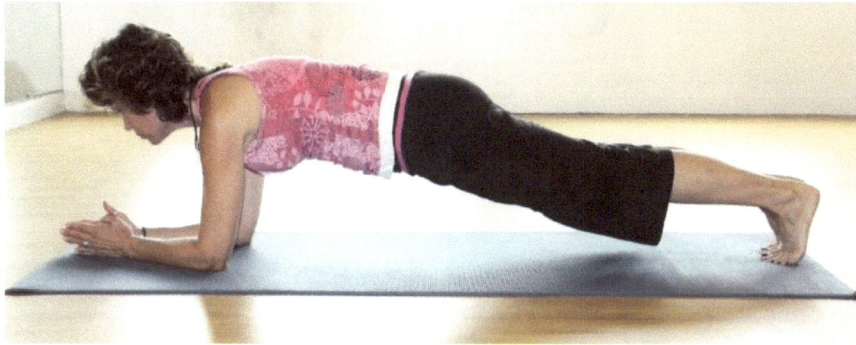

Plank on Elbows

With Belly Button Tucked to Spine

Momentary Sivasana

This Pose Can Be Repeated

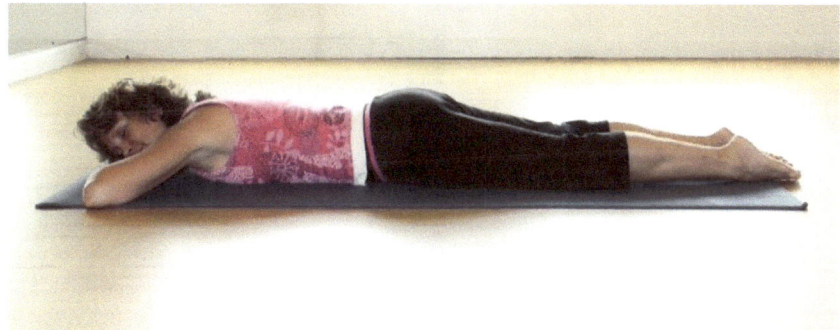

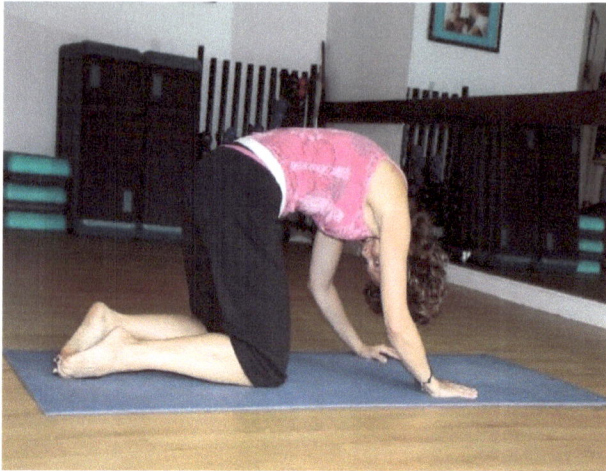

Cat to Cow

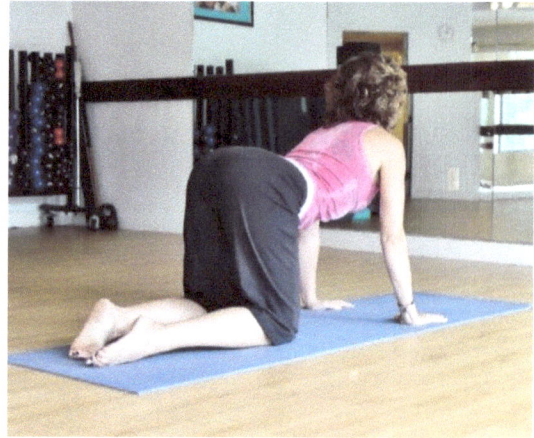

Down Dog

Tuck Belly Button in, Lift Tail to Sky and Lower Heels Towards Earth

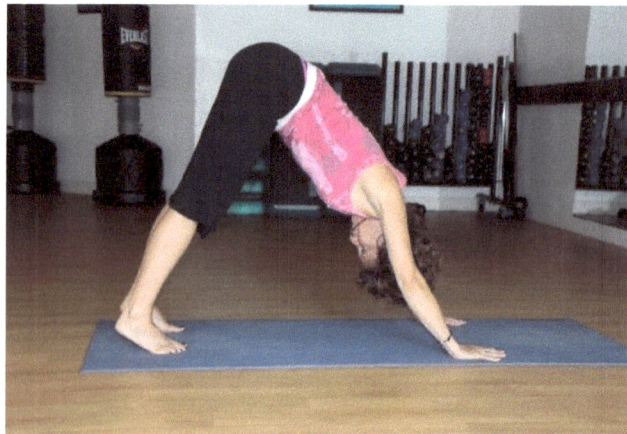

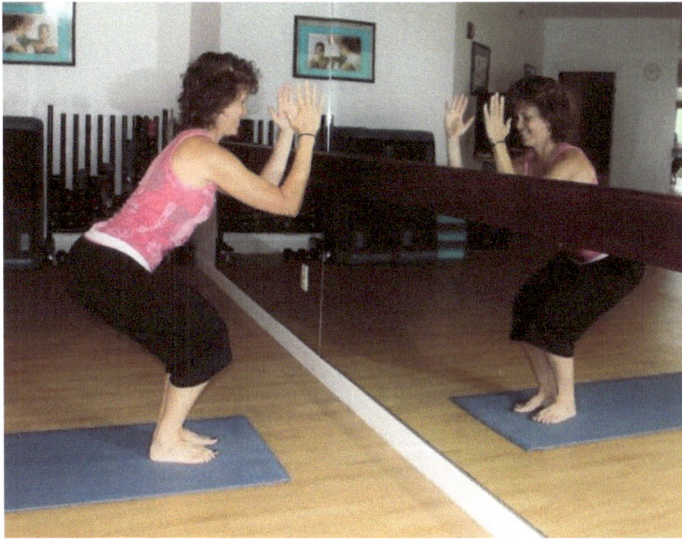

Chair

Tuck Your Belly Button in, Lower Sit bones as You Bend Knees

Chair with Twist

Complete on Each Side

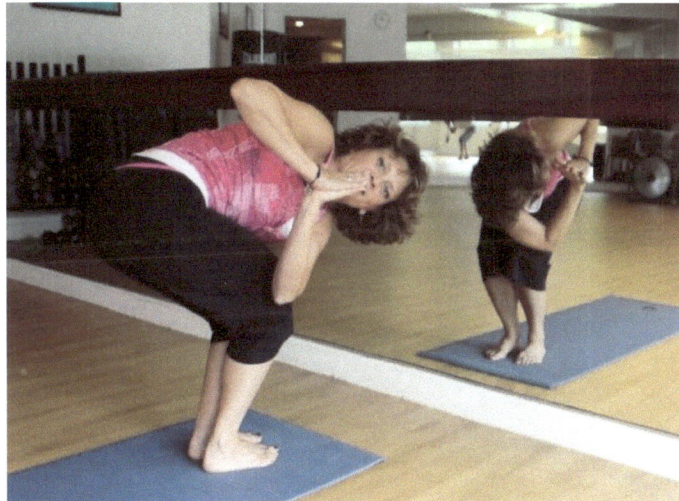

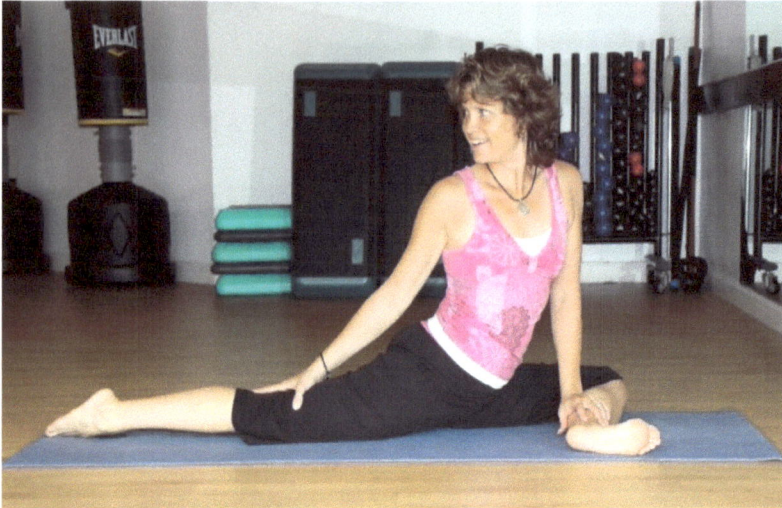

Partial Pigeon

Bend Front Leg, Open Chest and Rotate Back Leg Over onto Hip

Pigeon

Tuck Belly Button in as You Rotate Your Open Chest Down to Earth

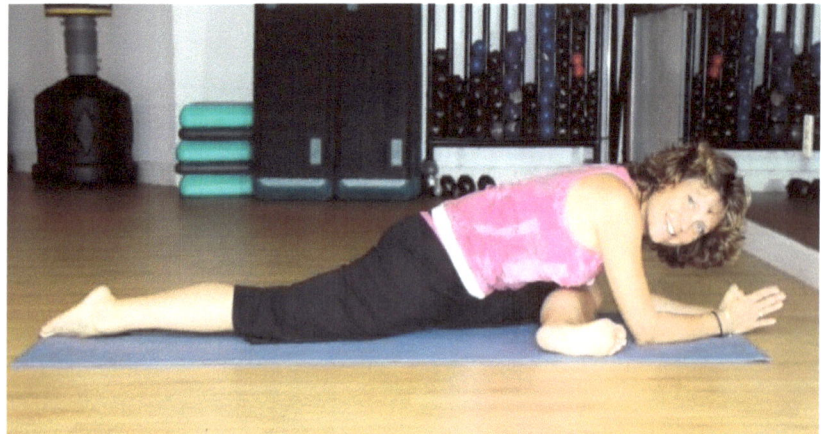

Complete on Each Side

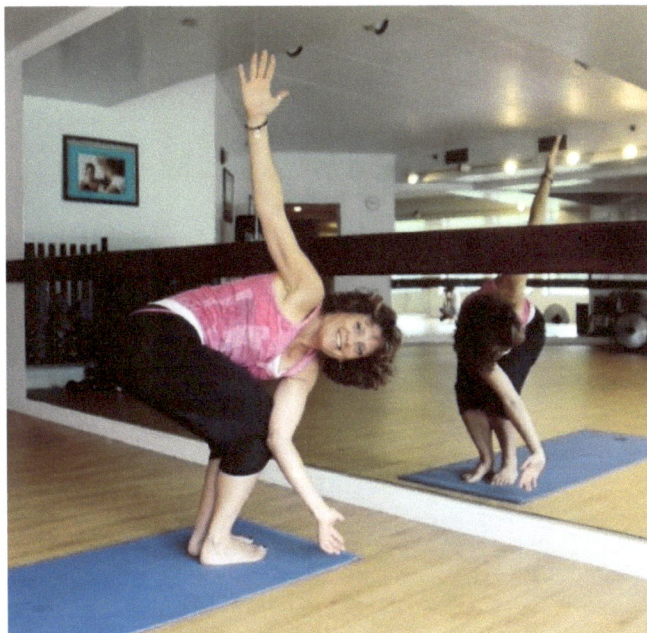

Chair with Twist

Extend Wing Span from the Earth to the Sky

Back to Chair

Complete on Each Side

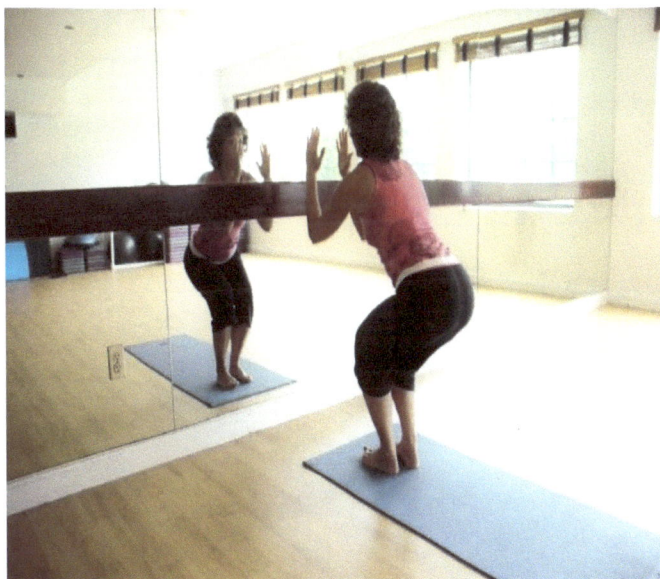

Partial Tree
on Left Side

**Place Foot on Ankle,
Calf or Thigh
Not at the Knee**

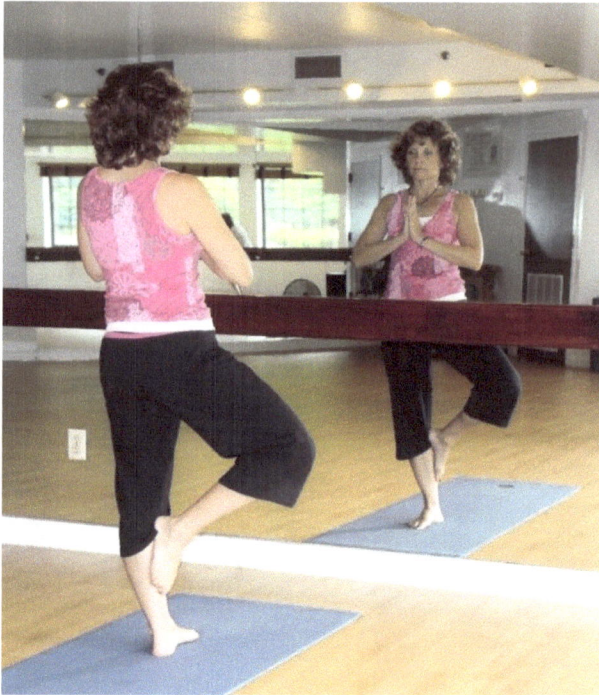

Tree Extend to
the Sky

**Engage From Waist to
Create Strong Trunk**

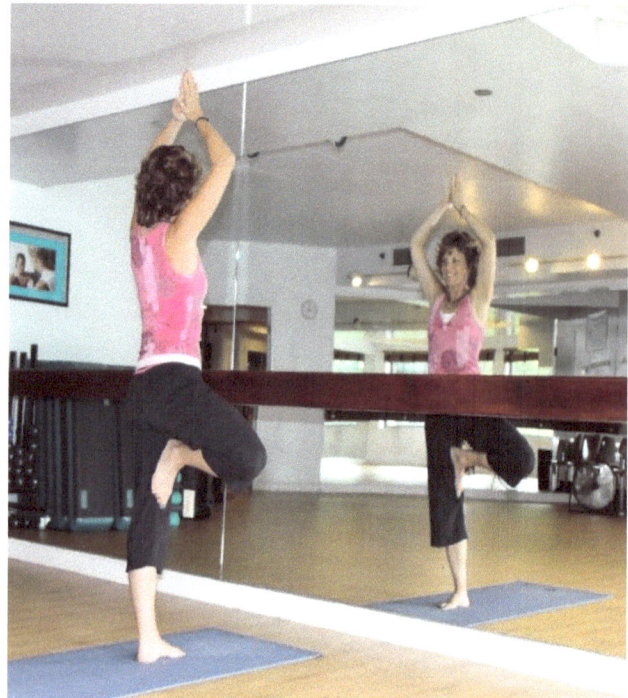

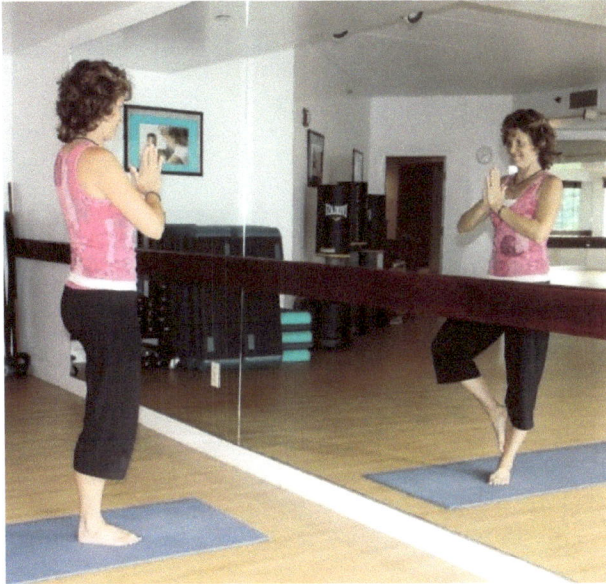

Partial Tree on Right Side

Place Foot on Ankle, Calf or Thigh Not at the Knee

Tree Extend to the Sky

Engage From Waist to Create Strong Trunk

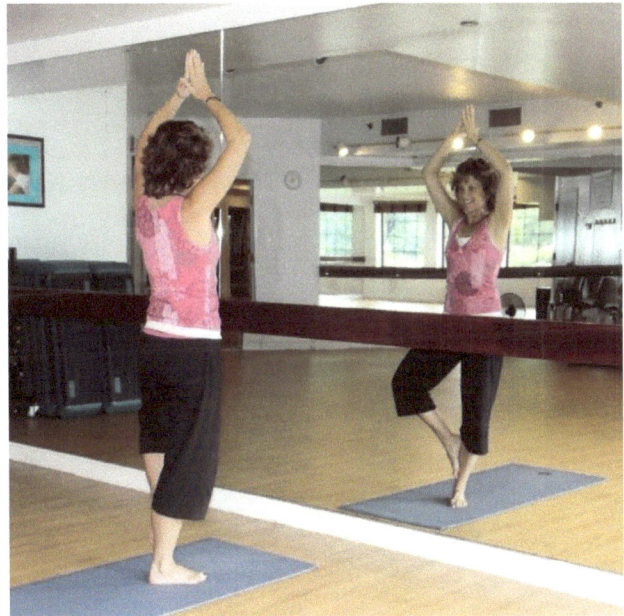

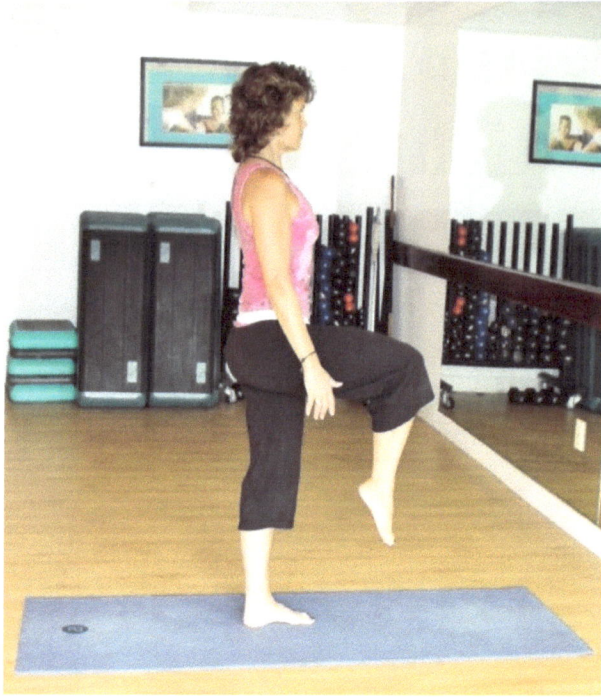

Left Leg
Balance
with Right
Knee Bent

With Arm
Extension

Complete on Each Side

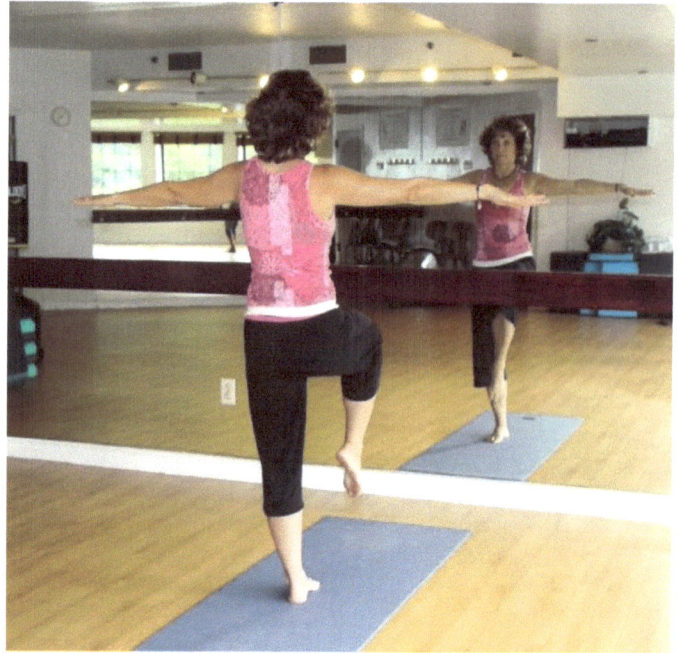

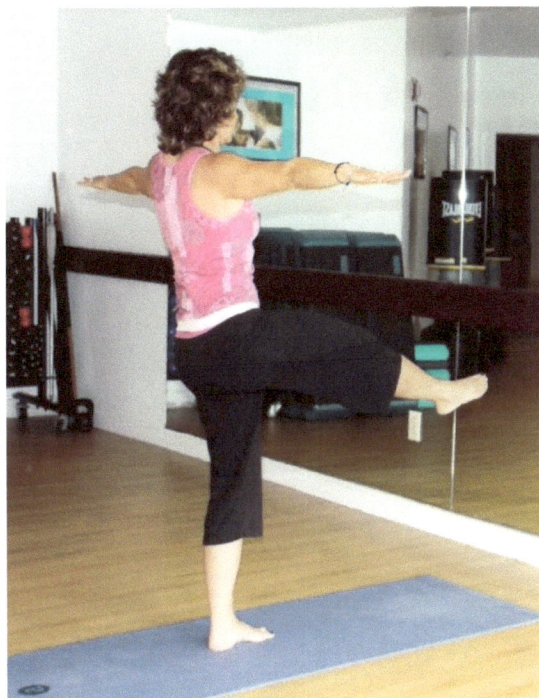

Full Extension to Front on Left

Rotate Right Leg Back

Warrior 3

With Chest Open, Arms Extended Straight & Belly Button Tucked In

Complete on Each Side

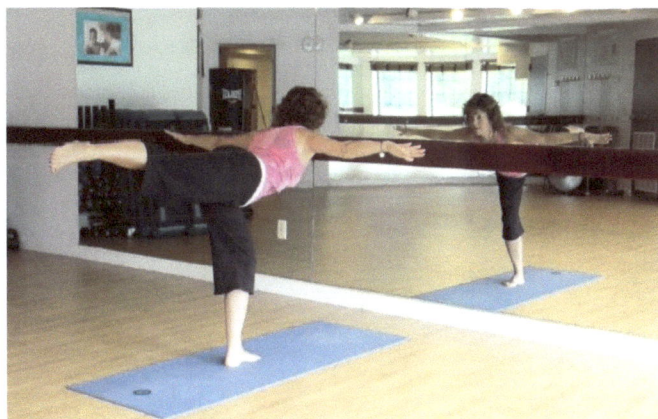

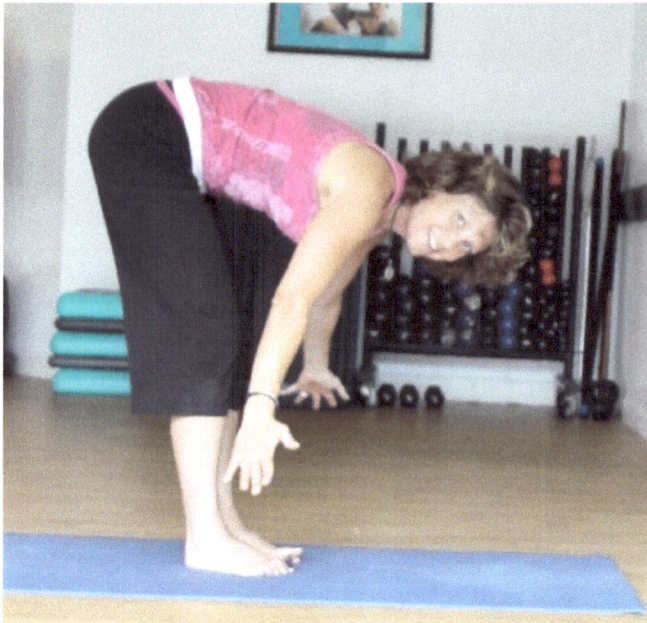

Forward Bend

Tuck Belly Button in as You Fold Chest to the Earth

Lift to Flat Back

Tuck the Belly Button In, Arms Extend Back with Chest Open and Crown of the Head to the Sky

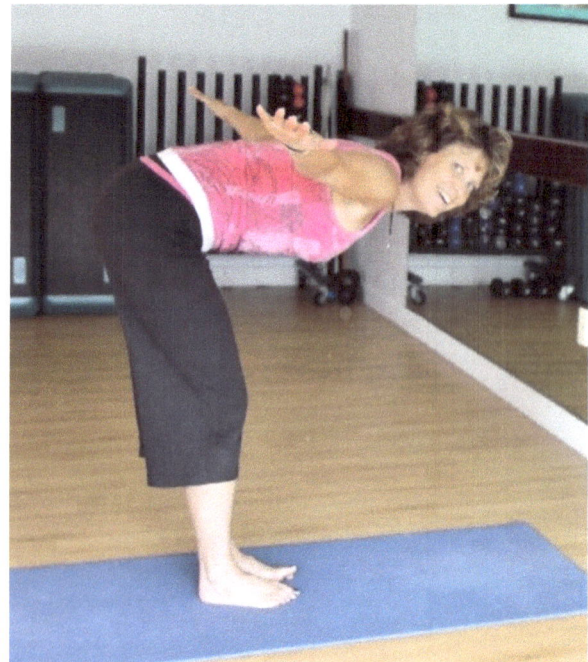

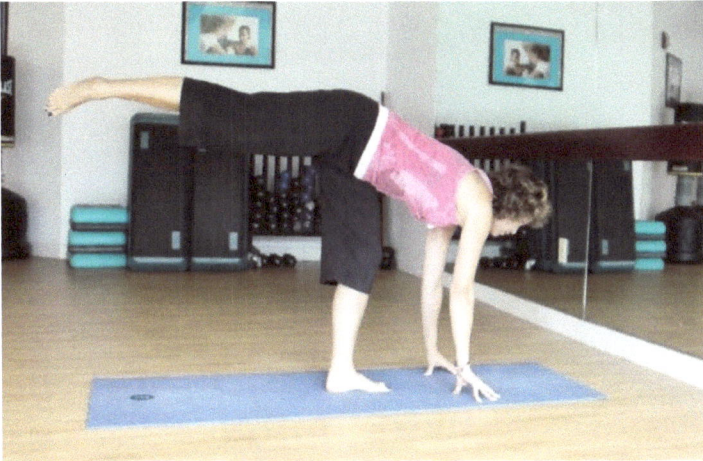

Forward Bend on Left Leg

Extend Arms to the Earth with Chest Open

Lift Right Arm

Or Both Arms Lift Up for More Advanced Asana

Complete on Each Side

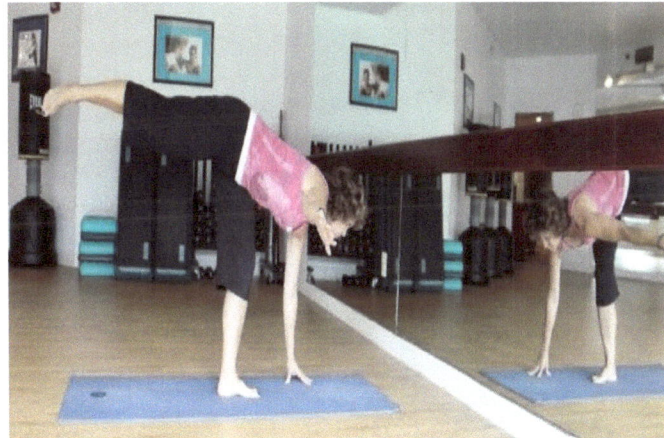

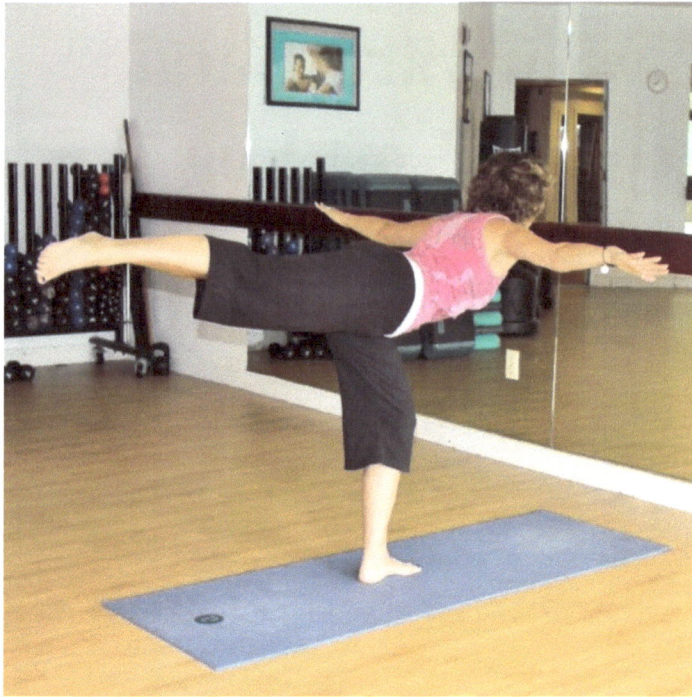

Warrior 3

With Chest Open, Arms Extended Straight & Belly Button Tucked In

With Hands to Ankle or Shin

For More Advanced Asana

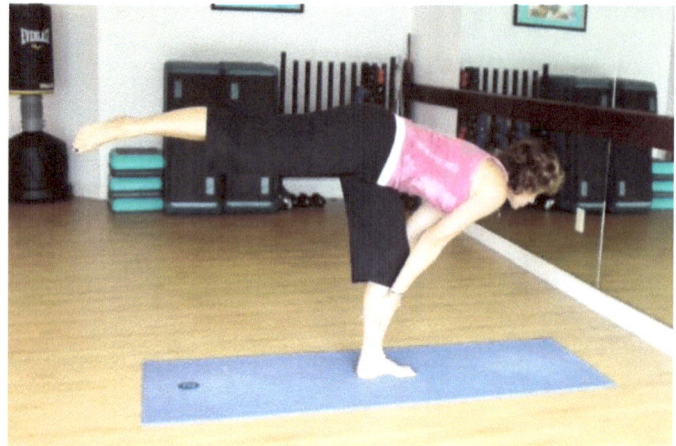

Complete on Each Side

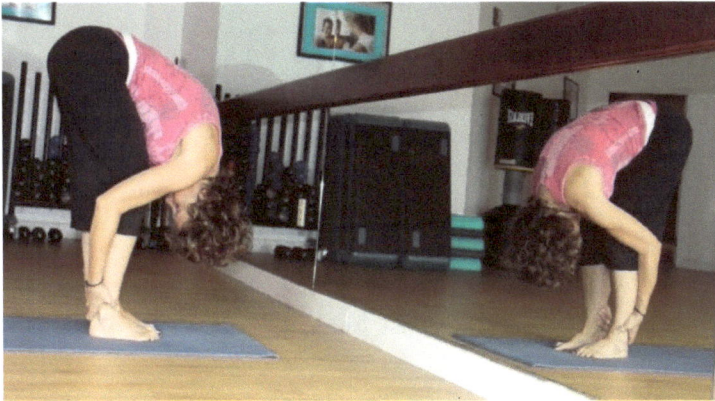

Forward Fold

With Arms and Palms Up to Flat Back

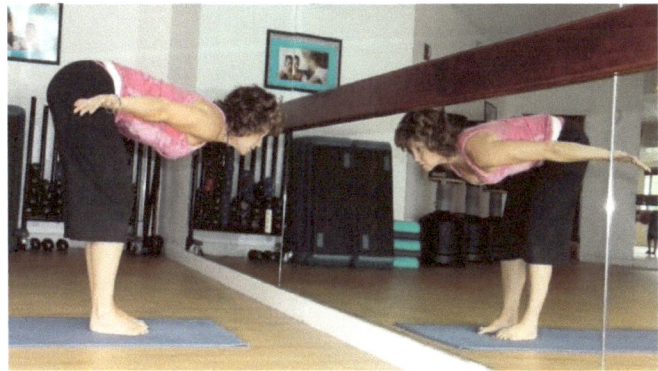

Rotate Back to Forward Fold Lift Hands to the Sky As You Lower Crown of Your Head

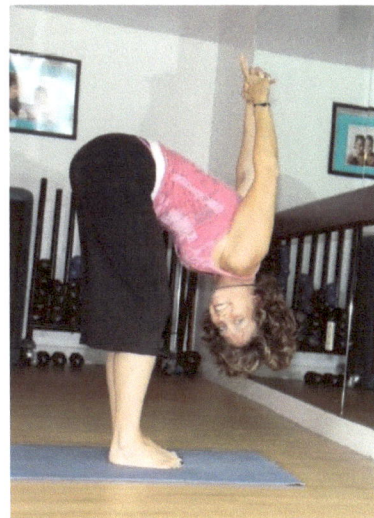

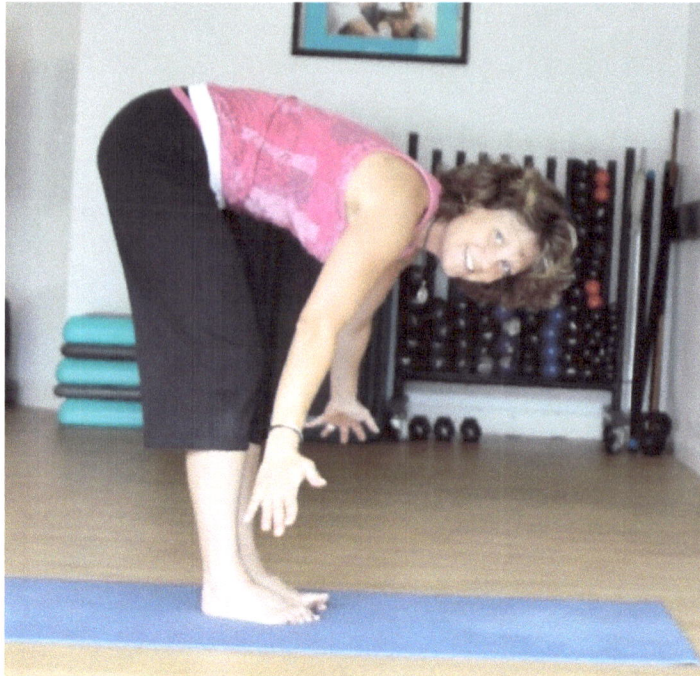

Stand Straight
First
Swan Dive
Down
to the Earth

Rotate Back
into Chair

Then Lower Down
to the Earth

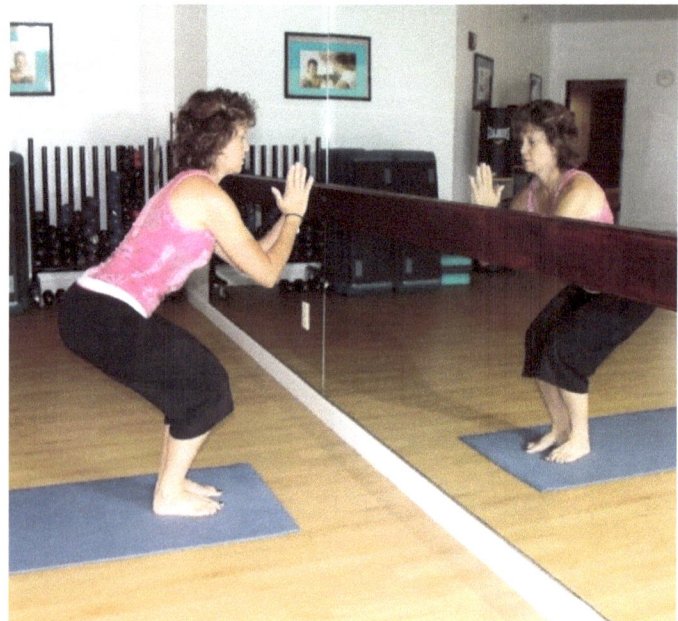

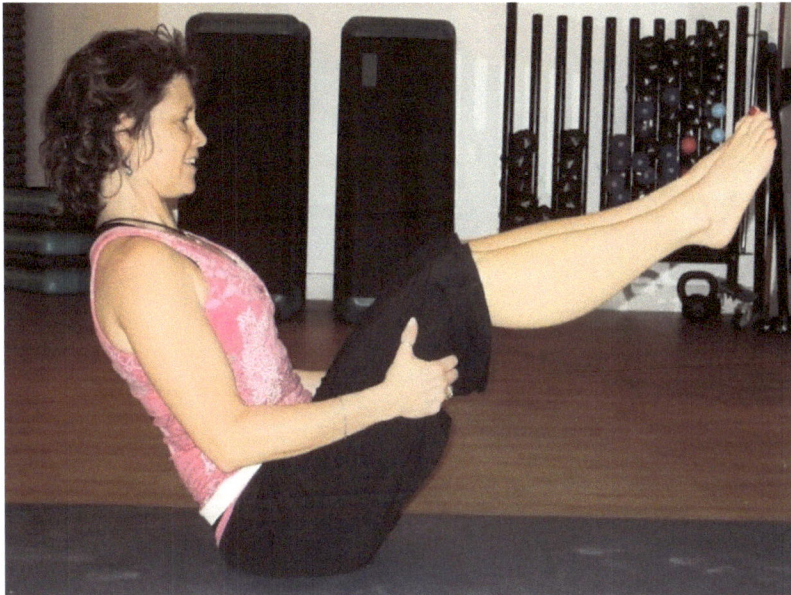

Boat

with Hands Support Modification

Full Boat

With Arms Extended And Belly Button Tucked into Spine

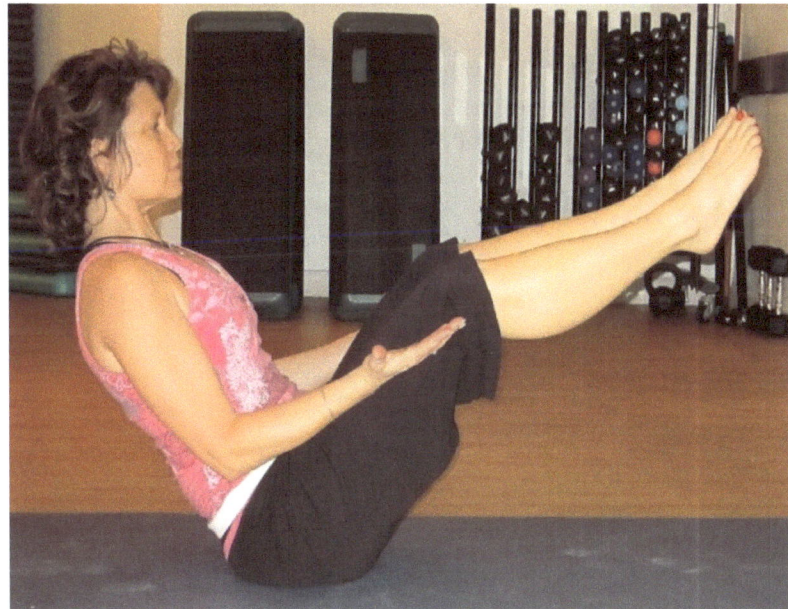

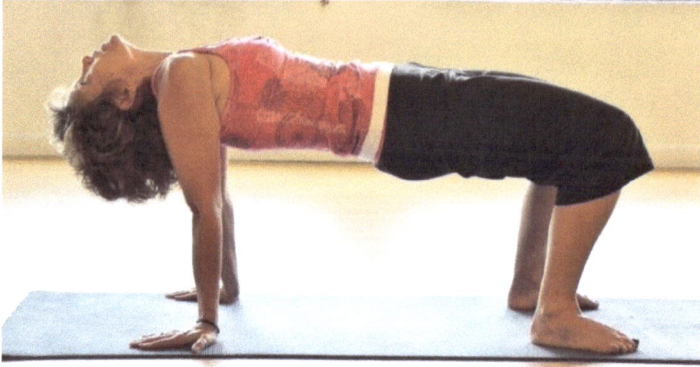

Table

Lift from Sit Bones to Flat Back with Chest Open

Table with One Arm Extended

For the Advanced Asana or Repeat Table

Complete on Each Side

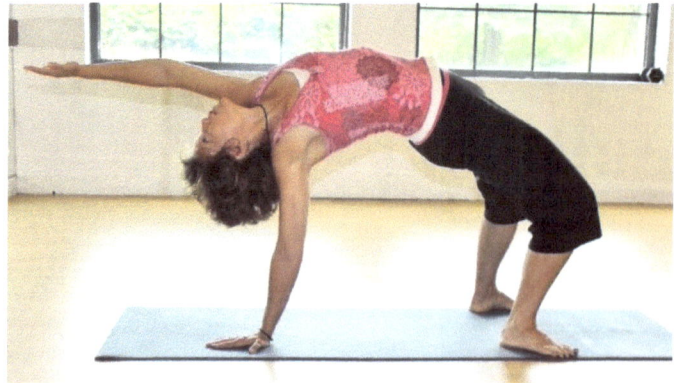

Reverse Plank

**Extend Arms Back
and Legs Out with
Toes Pointed,
Chest Open and
Hips Lifted to Sky**

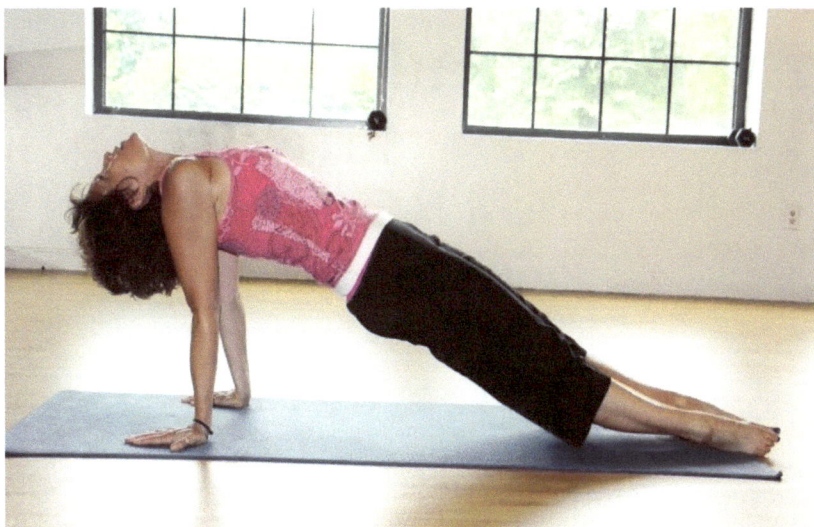

Side Plank
on Elbow

**Align Arm Under
Shoulder
Lift Hip as
You Tuck Belly Button In
to Spine**

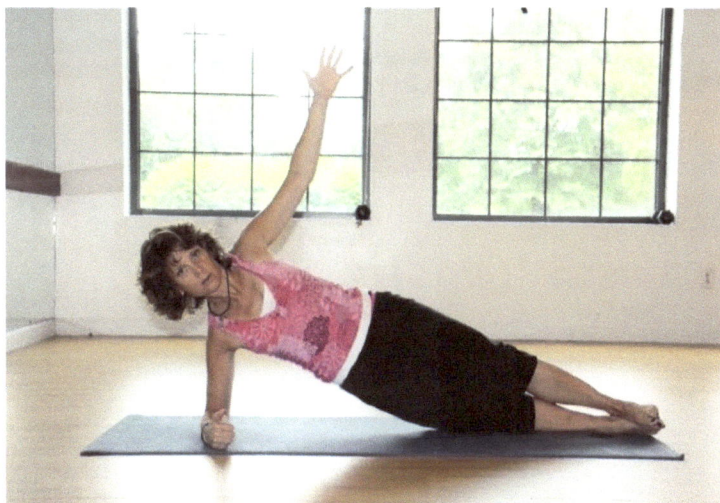

Complete on Each Side

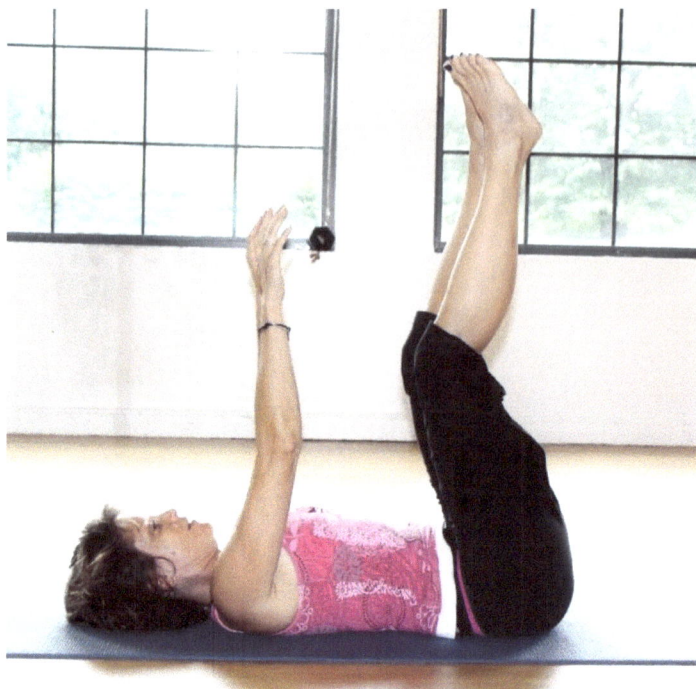

Dead Bug

Allow Head, Neck & Spine to Release to Earth While You Extend Arms & Legs to the Sky

Happy Baby

Fold Knees and Elbows Into your Center with Flat Back as You Open Chest and Hips

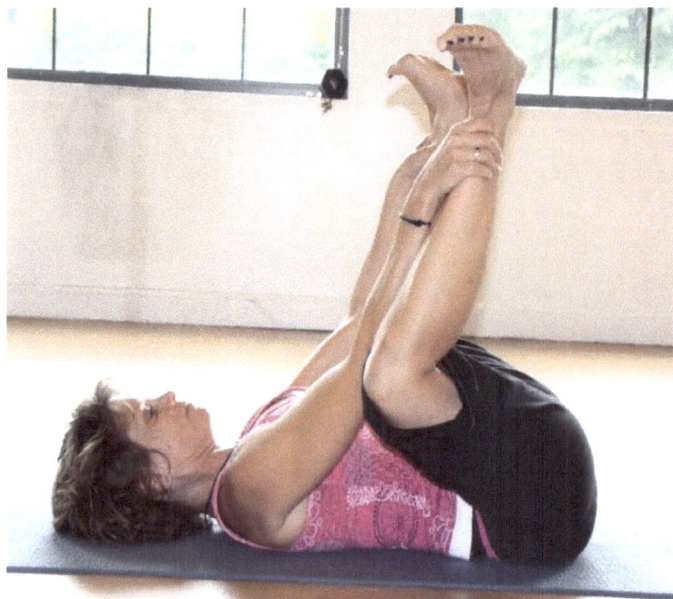

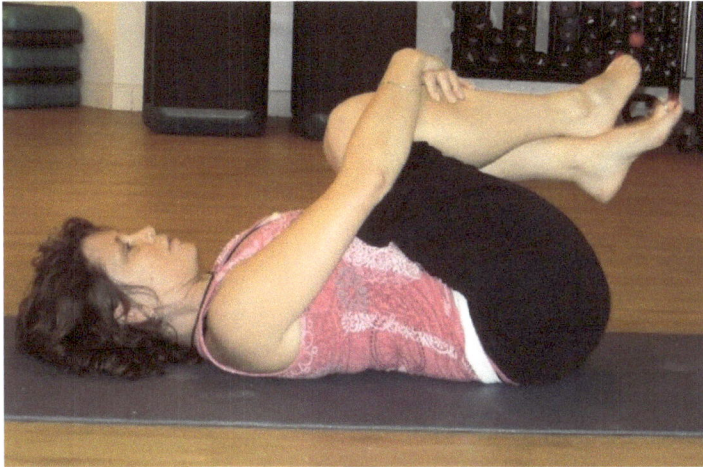

Ball

Visual You Have a Checkerboard on Your Back & Roll Side to Side Touching Each Square on Back to the Mat

Stretch to Toes

Extending Hands to Your Shins or Ankles with Back Pressed to the Mat and Stretch Legs

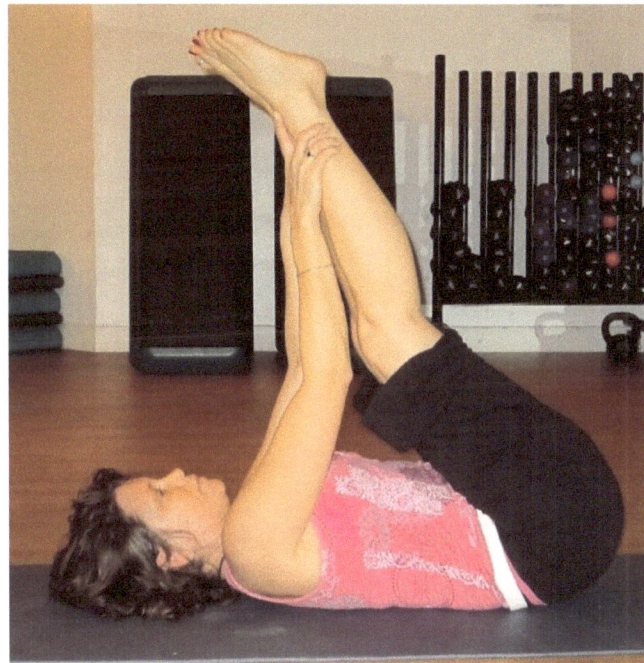

*These are Advanced Asanas. Partial Poses or Modifications May Be Utilized for Safety

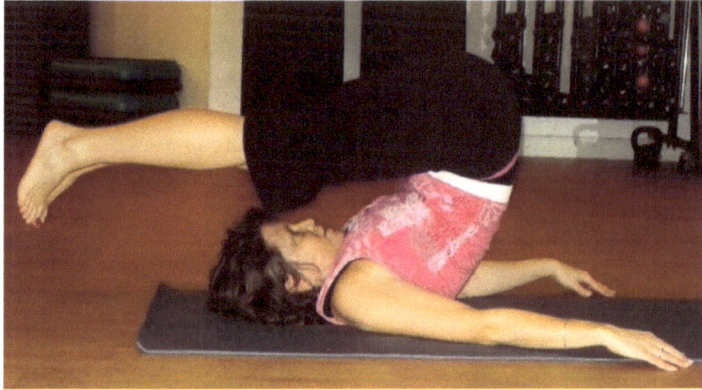

*Plough

Keep Your Nose Pointing Centered to Sky. Do Not Look Left or Right

*Shoulder Stand

Nose & Toes to the Sky Tuck Your Belly Button to Spine

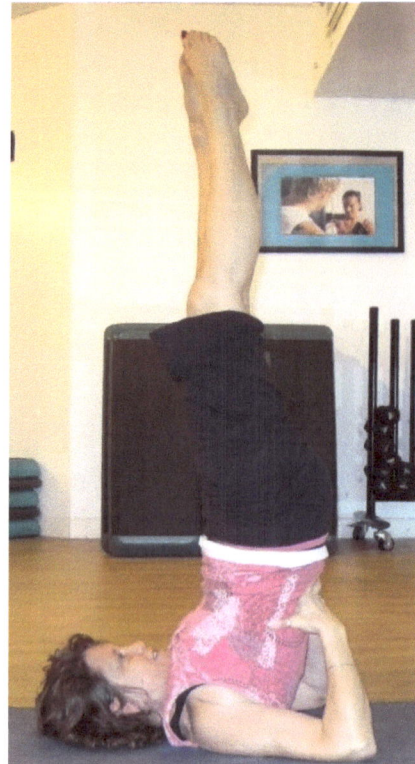

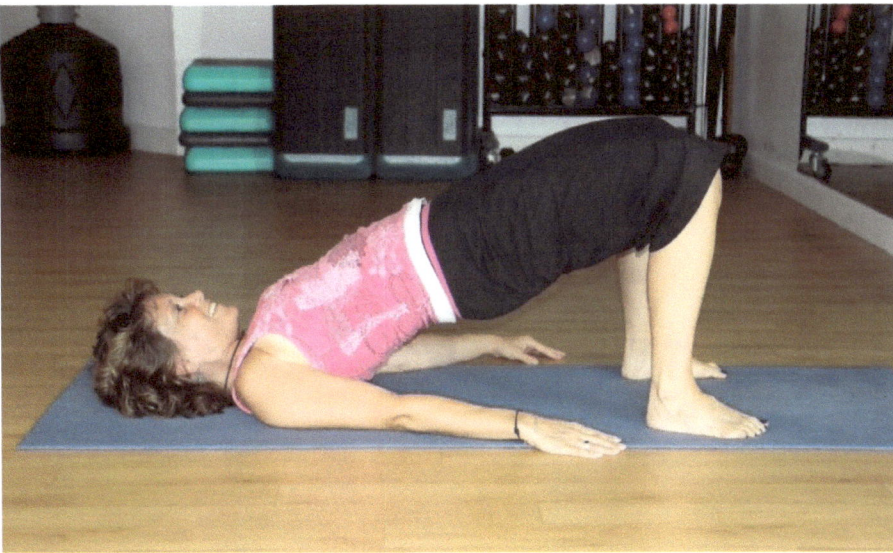

Bridge

Bend Knees Hip Distance Apart and Lift Hips With Belly Tucked to Sky with Open Chest

Release

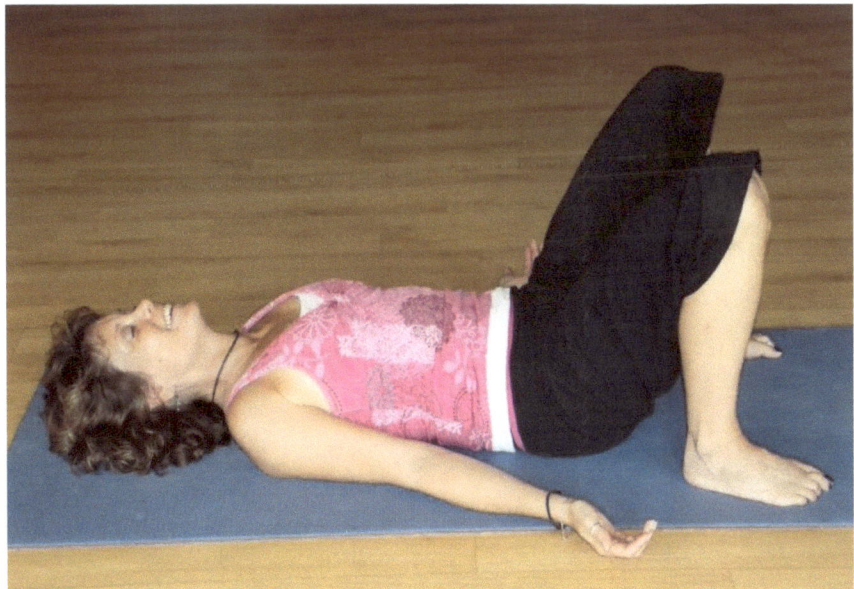

Allow Entire Body from Head to Tail to Drift Into the Earth As Your Full Body Relaxes

Spinal Twist to Left

Fold Right Leg In, Cross It over to the Left side as You Twist to the Right

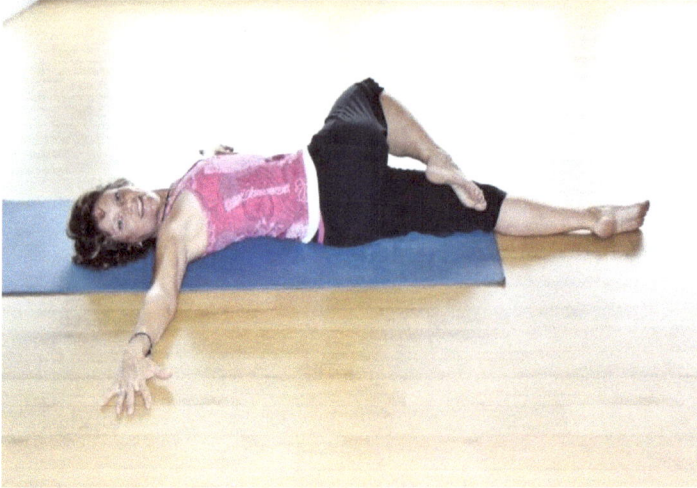

Spinal Twist to Right

Fold Left Leg In, Cross It over to the Right Side as You Twist to the Left

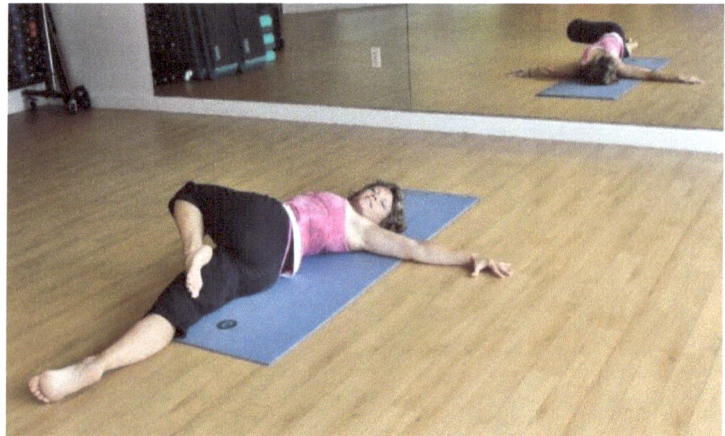

Savasana

FINAL RESTING POSE or the
Corpse position.

At the end of your daily practice you
will lay down supine on your mat and
work on your final asana. This should
be done with your eyes closed as you
retreat inward and revert your focus
back to your breath. Your heart rate
will slow as you quiet your mind.

Think about what you have achieved
in your practice and what you might
like to aspire to in the weeks ahead as
you drift. Acknowledge your thoughts
and then set them aside until deep
inner strength and harmony are
achieved.

See Next Page for Your Positioning

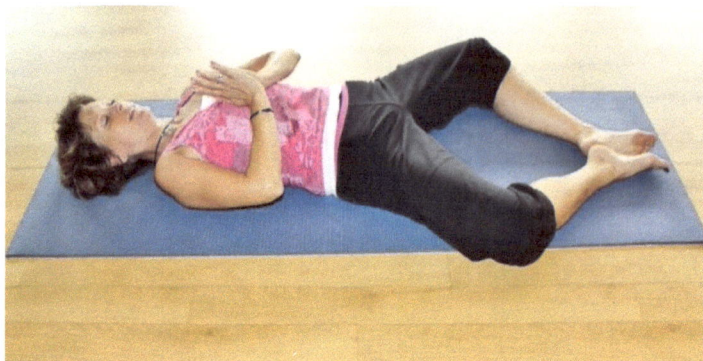

Final Resting Pose at Prayer

Corpse Position

**Your Choice or Move
from One Pose to the Other as
Your Body Releases to the Earth
and Your Mind Retreats
Until You Achieve**

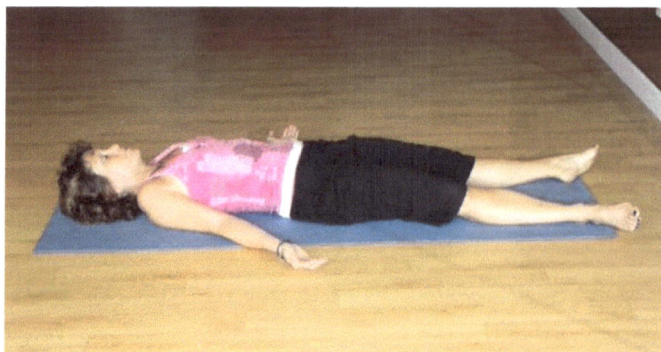

Deep Inner Strength

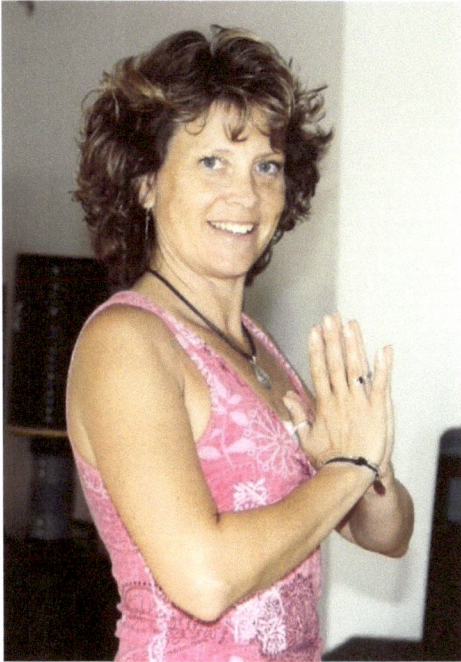

Namaste

The Light Inside Me

To The Light Inside of You

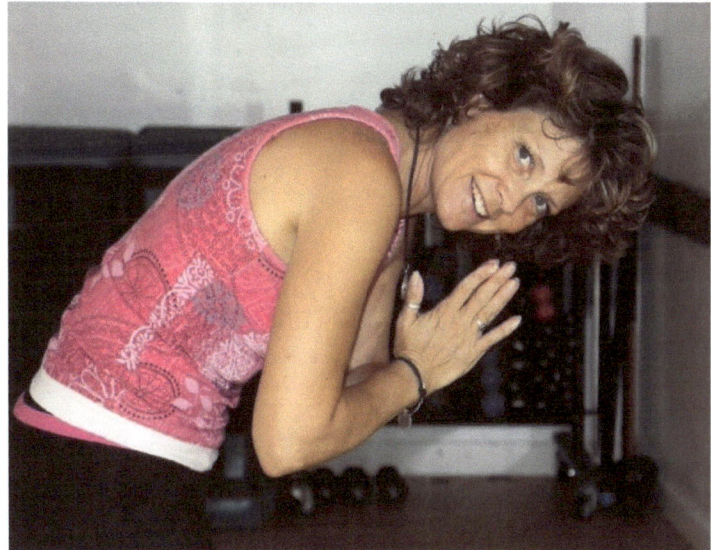

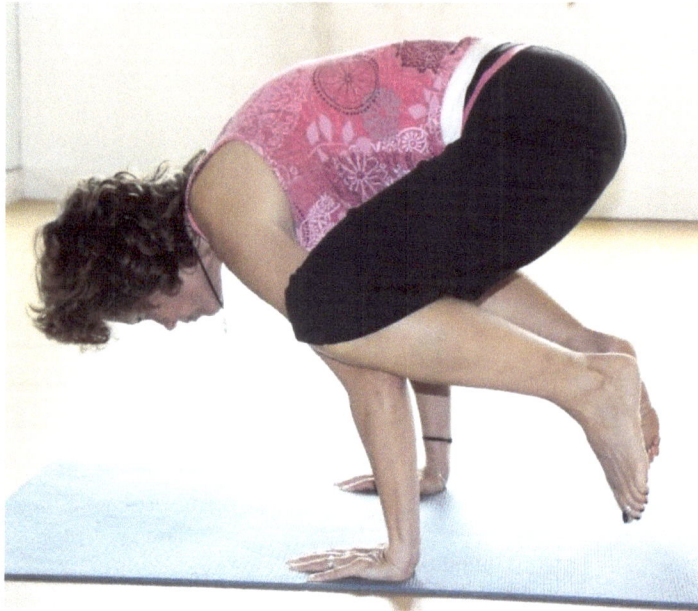

*Crane

*Wheel

*These Advanced
Asanas Are in This
Book to Inspire You
to Achieve More in
Your Practice.
It Will Come…

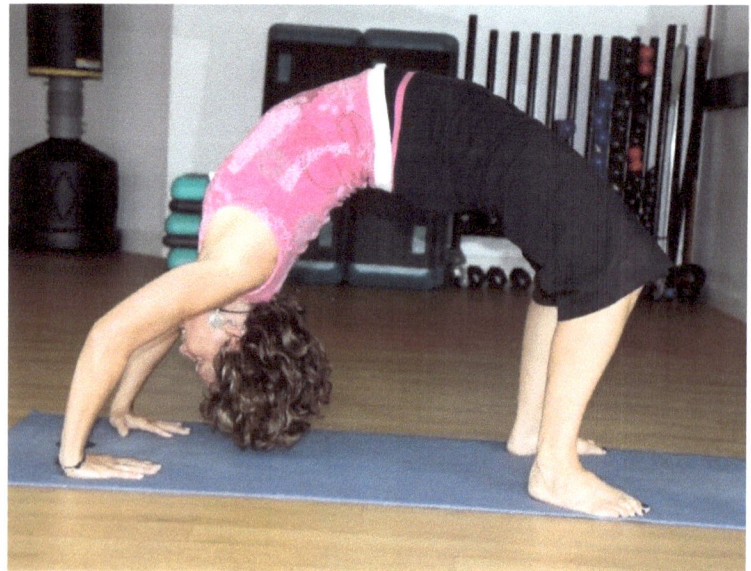

www.ingramcontent.com/pod-product-compliance
Lightning Source LLC
Chambersburg PA
CBHW060816270326
41930CB00002B/61